Training for Speed, Agility, and Quickness

Lee E. Brown
Vance A. Ferrigno
Juan Carlos Santana

Editors

Human Kinetics

Library of Congress Cataloging-in-Publication Data

Training for speed, agility, and quickness / Lee E. Brown, Vance Ferrigno, Juan Carlos
  Santana, editors.
     p.   cm.
  ISBN 0-7360-0239-1
     1. Physical education and training. 2. Speed. 3. Motor ability. 4. Coaching (Athletics)
  I. Brown, Lee E., 1956- II. Ferrigno, Vance, 1961- III. Santana, Juan Carlos, 1959-

GV711.5 .S64 2000
613.7'11--dc   99-0088413
                                                                                     CIP
ISBN: 0-7360-0239-1

This book and the drills herein are in no way associated with or endorsed by SAQ INTER-
NATIONAL and are not representative of SAQ Programmes. This book does not reflect the
subject matter of SAQ Accreditation Awards and is not approved for use by SAQ Trainers.

Developmental Editor: Kent Reel; **Assistant Editor:** Kim Thoren; **Copyeditor:** Harbour
Hodder; **Proofreader:** Sue Fetters; **Graphic Designer:** Robert Reuther; **Graphic Artist:** Kim
Maxey; **Cover Designer:** Jack W. Davis; **Photographer (cover and interior):** Tom Roberts;
Illustrator: Roberto Sabas, **Art Manager:** Craig Newsom; **Printer:** United Graphics

Human Kinetics books are available at special discounts for bulk purchase. Special editions or
book excerpts can also be created to specification. For details, contact the Special Sales
Manager at Human Kinetics.

Printed in the United States of America   10   9

Human Kinetics
Web site: www.HumanKinetics.com

United States: Human Kinetics, P.O. Box 5076, Champaign, IL 61825-5076
800-747-4457
e-mail: humank@hkusa.com

Canada: Human Kinetics, 475 Devonshire Road, Unit 100, Windsor, ON N8Y 2L5
800-465-7301 (in Canada only)
e-mail: orders@hkcanada.com

Europe: Human Kinetics, 107 Bradford Road, Stanningley
Leeds LS28 6AT, United Kingdom
+44 (0) 113 255 5665
e-mail: hk@hkeurope.com

Australia: Human Kinetics, 57A Price Avenue, Lower Mitcham, South Australia 5062
08 8277 1555
e-mail: liaw@hkaustralia.com

New Zealand: Human Kinetics, Division of Sports Distributors NZ Ltd.
P.O. Box 300 226 Albany, North Shore City, Auckland
0064 9 448 1207
e-mail: blairc@hknewz.com

To the unsung heroes and their support ...
Theresa, Ann-Marie and Debbie.

Contents

Preface

How does a coach increase the athletic performance of his players? That is the question answered by this book of drills. The following pages contain a collection of drills you can use to assist your players in their quest for speed, agility, and quickness. The quest to improve athletic performance within the ever-shrinking time limits placed on the coach is an ongoing challenge. In addition, misleading information or complicated formulas can sometimes muddy the waters when it comes to choosing exercises for a team. This book will focus on a straightforward approach to implementing drills for the coach and player alike. These drills are not standard-issue weight-room exercises but rather nontraditional field drills that can be used at minimal expense.

The motive for this book was akin to most innovations in sports today: that is, necessity is the mother of invention. After conducting field demonstrations of the drills in this book at a National Strength and Conditioning Association (NSCA) Florida State clinic, we were flooded with requests for an easy-to-use compilation of drills. This book is the answer to those requests.

We have designed this book so that it can be read from front to back or back to front, depending on the reader's experience with coaching and training. The first chapter concentrates on proper preparation for speed, agility, and quickness exercise by explaining equipment, warm-up, basic muscle physiology, and human performance. Next is a chapter on needs analysis, which focuses on preparing your athletes for training by first performing the proper testing and assessment required to properly evaluate the need for a speed, agility, and quickness program.

The middle section contains the real essence of the book. These three chapters (speed, agility, and quickness) contain all the drills, simply stated for quick implementation by the coach. There are pictures and instructions for each drill, making them accessible at a glance.

The final chapter is designed for the introductory reader. Here, a full complement of drills are explained and chosen to address many unique sporting activities. These include basketball, football, baseball, tennis, and others. This chapter utilizes case studies to illustrate how the coach might interject drills into a comprehensive strength and conditioning program.

As editors, we have attempted to design a book that can be carried in the coach's bag and used at a moment's notice. Additionally, the book can be studied at home and used to implement safe and effective long- and short-term strength and conditioning programs. We hope you enjoy reading it as much as we enjoyed writing it.

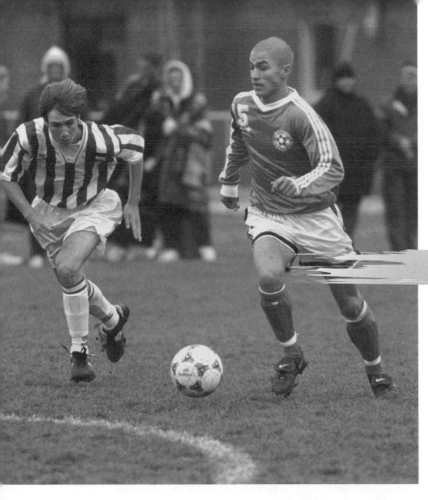

Introduction to Speed, Agility, and Quickness Training

Lee E. Brown, EdD, CSCS, *D

Joshua M. Miller, MS, NSCA-CPT

Jim Roberts, MS, CSCS

Speed, agility, and quickness training has become a popular way to train athletes. Whether they are school children on a soccer field or professionals in a training camp, they can all benefit from speed, agility, and quickness training. This method has been around for several years, but it is not used by all athletes primarily due to a lack of education regarding the drills. Speed, agility, and quickness training may be used to increase speed or strength, or the ability to exert maximal force during high-speed movements. It manipulates and capitalizes on the stretch-shortening cycle while bridging the gap between traditional resistance training and functional-specific movements. Some benefits of speed, agility, and quickness training include increases in muscular power in all multiplanar movements; brain signal efficiency; kinesthetic or body spatial awareness; motor skills; and reaction time.

Speed, agility, and quickness training can cover the complete spectrum of training intensity, from low to high intensity. Every individual will come into a training program at a different level; thus training intensities must coincide with the individual's abilities. Low intensity speed, agility, and quickness drills can be used by everyone for different applications. For example, the assorted biomotor skills illustrated throughout this book can be used to teach movement, warmup, or condition any athlete. No significant preparation is needed to participate at this level of speed, agility, and quickness training. Higher intensity drills require a significant level of preparation. A simple approach to safe participation and increased effectiveness is to start a concurrent strength training program when starting speed, agility, and quickness training.

Coaches will be able to use this reference in whole or in part for their desired sport. It has been designed to examine each section of speed, agility, and quickness training and assist the coach in writing a program that will be sport-specific.

BASIC MUSCLE PHYSIOLOGY

This section provides a brief overview of how muscles work to create forces across joints that result in movement. Understanding the basic physiology of the muscle will be invaluable in writing a speed, agility, and quickness training program.

Each skeletal muscle is made up of connective tissue, muscle tissue, nerves, and blood vessels and is controlled by signals sent from the brain. These components work together in a coordinated fashion to cause bones and therefore limbs to move in desired patterns. Muscle tissue is connected to a tendon that is a noncontractile length of tissue that connects the muscle to a bone. Thus tension developed within the muscle results in that tension being transferred to the adjoining tendon and then the bone.

Within each muscle fiber are hundreds to thousands of thin longitudinal fibers. Within these fibers are two opposing, contractile, fingerlike proteins called actin and myosin. These fibers form attachments called cross-bridges and pull against one another to cause motion. Through a series of chemical reactions that are regulated via brain signals, these proteins work to repeatedly pull and release, causing muscular work or a contraction to occur.

STRETCH-SHORTENING CYCLE

The stretch-shortening cycle (SSC) is described as the combination of eccentric (muscle-lengthening) and concentric (muscle-shortening) actions. An eccentric muscle action is performed when an athlete lowers a weight, such as in the down portion of the movement in a biceps curl or a squat exercise. A concentric muscle action is the upward motion or opposite movement during the above exercises. When an eccentric action precedes a concentric action, the resulting force output of the concentric action is increased. The stretch-shortening cycle works like a rubber band that is stretched and then snaps back together. This is the essence of the stretch-shortening cycle and speed, agility, and quickness training. Examples in sports are a baseball or golf swing where an athlete precedes the intended motion with a wind-up or prestretch. Without the eccentric action, or if there is a pause between the two actions, the increased force output of the concentric phase of the exercise will not occur. The stretch-shortening cycle takes place during everyday activities such as walking and running, yet it is intensified greatly during speed, agility, and quickness training.

Advantages derived from the stretch-shortening cycle can be seen in sports competition. One example is a normal vertical jump. When the jumper precedes her jump by bending at the knees and hips and then explodes upward, the resultant jump height will be greater than when performing the same movement by stopping at the bottom for a few seconds before the explosion portion of the jump. Another example can be seen in the baseball throw. If the thrower does not complete a wind-up, he would be unable to generate as much force as he would by performing a prestretch motion.

Stretch-shortening cycle activities can be done for the upper body as well as for the lower body and can be implemented with external devices such as free weights, rubber tubing, and medicine balls. Devices such as these assist the athlete in performing both the concentric and eccentric portions of the exercise due to the need to either accelerate or decelerate the object. However, speed, agility, and quickness training may be performed without assisting devices by simply using one's own body mass as the weight or resistance.

MUSCLE SORENESS AND PERIODIZATION

It is a common experience that when an athlete attempts a new exercise there may be an occurrence of muscle soreness. This soreness, or more specifically "delayed onset muscle soreness (DOMS)," usually peaks between 24 and 36 hours after the exercise bout. The eccentric or lengthening portion of the exercise primarily causes DOMS. Currently, the prevailing explanation for DOMS is micro-muscle tears. This has been observed in studies utilizing an electron microscope to reveal tissue damage in the fibers. The only way to reduce the development of

DOMS is to "adapt" to the exercise stress. This requires repeated exercise bouts over several weeks with sufficient rest between sessions. Since all speed, agility, and quickness training involves eccentric exercise utilizing the stretch-shortening cycle, it is recommended that no more than two exercise sessions per week separated by two or three days be employed with novice athletes.

Periodization is the gradual cycling of frequency, intensity, and volume of training to achieve peak levels of fitness for the most important competitions. Periodization organizes training into cycles of training objectives, tasks, and content. The overall training cycle usually refers to the entire training year but may be separated into smaller more manageable sections. These time cycles may last from weeks to months, depending upon the goals set by the athlete. Each cycle contains a number of microcycles, which are generally periods of one week of training. The cycle may also depend upon the type of athletic event being prepared for.

GETTING STARTED

An appropriate warm-up session should precede every exercise session. Warm-up routines should begin with a general whole body activity such as cycling, walking, or jogging at a low intensity. This will increase heat and blood flow to the muscles and tendons, thereby preparing them for higher intensity workouts. This general warm-up should be followed by a specific warm-up that would consist of performing some of the session's exercises at a low intensity.

Injury prevention is a major part of any exercise program. It is imperative that one follows proper progression when embarking on any program, including speed, agility, and quickness training. A strength training program that emphasizes knee, hip, back, and ankle strength will reduce the possibility of injury when speed, agility, and quickness training is first introduced. Similar to a traditional resistance-training program, speed, agility, and quickness training should be progressive and systematic in nature. Training should progress from simple to complex movements, from low to high intensity, and from gross to sport-specific motor patterns. Factors such as frequency, intensity, volume, body structure, sport specificity, training age, and time in relation to one's season should be considered when designing an speed, agility, and quickness training program. The following are a few recommendations for injury prevention:

- Follow the proper progression of exercises.
- Perform one or more warm-up sets with no resistance or a very light resistance.
- Perform all exercises through a complete range of motion.
- Wear proper clothing and shoes. No bare feet or thongs, and no jeans or constrictive clothing.

Proper safety procedures must be observed while learning and mastering the speed, agility, and quickness activities included in this book. Make certain that all equipment is in correct working order before use. If you are exercising outdoors, make sure the area is free from any hazardous objects such as rocks or trees. Be sure to understand each new exercise completely before attempting it for the first time.

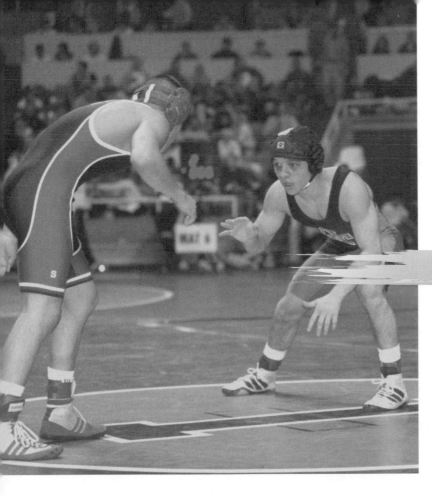

Needs Analysis

Steven Scott Plisk, MS, CSCS

peed of execution and technical precision are fundamental athletic goals and are, of course, interrelated. Movement speed is the result of explosive force but is often incorrectly believed to be independent from—or incompatible with—strength. In fact, explosive speed-strength applied to functional motor skills is the basis for speed, agility, and quickness.

Running is the basis of many sports and has a ballistic quality common to other movements. However, most sports involve much more than linear sprinting at top speed. The ability to change direction and velocity is often more important. Changes in direction involve explosive braking actions that are executed by rapidly and forcibly lengthening the muscles. The inability to withstand such extreme stretch-loading, as it is called, can result in injury, technical inefficiency, and outright nonathleticism. This is especially important when considering that the body is alternately supported on one leg during speed, agility, and quickness maneuvers. It is, therefore, a serious error to focus one's testing and training exclusively on linear speed mechanics while neglecting decelerative mechanics and oblique angles of acceleration.

Changing speed and direction also requires the muscles to shorten in an elastic or reactive manner, immediately after lengthening. In this sense, many speed, agility, and quickness drills can be considered single-leg plyometric movements with horizontal emphasis. Therefore, reactive types of single-leg movements should be progressively addressed in conjunction with heavy-resistance training and testing.

Few athletic activities involve a single, brief effort. Most sports consist of ongoing activity with intense, intermittent bursts—or a series of plays with periodic rest. The athlete must have the specific metabolic power to execute his or her assignments at the requisite effort level—and the capacity (and recoverability) to do so repetitively. A simple way to address this is to model special-endurance training and testing on actual competition work/rest schemes. That is, you ultimately want to match your conditioning training to the demands of your sport. After speed, agility, and quickness skills are mastered, you can create a "game-like" environment in your speed, agility, and quickness training.

MOVEMENT MECHANICS

Most sport skills involve rapid force generation. As a case in point, force is applied for one to two seconds during many athletic tasks, whereas absolute maximum force production requires up to six to eight seconds.[15,18-20,25,28,32,37] Even in nonballistic movements, performance is usually determined by the ability to develop forces quickly and achieve a "critical power output" (velocity with given resistance).

Many movements have a reactive or ballistic nature regardless of whether they are initiated from a dynamic or static position. This phenomenon, referred to as the stretch-shortening cycle (SSC) and as defined in chapter 1, is especially prevalent in athletics.[16,19,20,25,26,28,31,37] SSC actions exploit the myotatic reflex as well as the elastic qualities of tendon and muscle, and the resulting performance is independent of maximum strength in elite athletes.[21,26,29] In contrast, the role of strength in determining movement speed increases with resistance.[4,18,19,25,26,28,33,34,37] The implications of this are obvious when considering that the mass of the athlete's body, equipment, or opponent must be overcome explosively—by a single support leg—during speed, agility, and quickness maneuvers.

These facts collectively illustrate that the evaluation of explosive strength is the starting point for determining the role of speed, agility, and quickness training in an athlete's preparation. Fortunately, such tests are relatively simple to administer and interpret.

ACTIVITY AND ATHLETE EVALUATION

A proper speed, agility, and quickness needs analysis involves three types of evaluation: the athlete's functional strength, his or her movement technique, and the specific metabolic demands of competition.

Functional Strength

The following is a four-pronged approach for evaluating an athlete's functional strength qualities: basic strength, reactive resources, strength deficit, and speed-strength. The first two methods are appropriate for novice or intermediate athletes, whereas the latter two should be used with discretion when progressing to more advanced levels.

Basic Strength   It is commonly proposed that athletes should be able to squat one and a half to two times their own body weight before undertaking "shock" types of plyometric training such as depth jumping.[14,28,29,36,37] Due to the fact that this criteria would eliminate most of the athletes we work with, we left depth jumps out of the drill. Furthermore, the ability to single-leg squat one's own body weight—as well as to lunge forward, laterally, or backward—with sound technique is also a useful prerequisite and more applicable to an introductory level. Such movements are also valuable in identifying and correcting bilateral strength imbalances.

Reactive Resources   Periodic measurement of reactive strength resources can be useful in determining an athlete's training status.[25,26] This involves comparing squat jump performance with drop jumps from heights of 16, 24, 32, 40, 48, and possibly 56 centimeters, depending on the qualification level of the athlete. A novice athlete's best drop-jump performance may be 20 to 25 percent below his or her squat jump, indicating large reactive resources. This can be interpreted as a functional deficit in short-response SSC abilities, with the subsequent need to emphasize reactive movements (such as drop jumps, vertical jumps, or countermovement jumps) in training. In contrast, an elite athlete's drop-jump result may be up to 20 to 25 percent greater than his or her squat jump, indicating small reactive resources. In this case, basic strength should be emphasized through hypertrophic or neural adaptations in order to create new reactive resources.

Strength Deficit   The eccentric-concentric strength deficit can be used to determine an advanced athlete's training status.[25,26,28,37] This indicates the difference between absolute involuntary (eccentric) strength and maximum voluntary (concentric) strength, and reflects the ability to use one's strength potential in a given motor task. Specifically, a large deficit (e.g., up to 45 percent) indicates that explosive methods should be emphasized in order to improve neuromuscular activation; whereas a small deficit (e.g., 5 percent) indicates that hypertrophic methods should be emphasized, followed by maximal heavy efforts.

Without force-plate equipment (expensive, specialized equipment that measures the amount of force exerted by a muscle), maximal eccentric strength measurement can be problematic, because muscles can sustain up to 30 to 40 percent greater loads while lengthening when compared with shortening. As a practical solution, eccentric strength can be approximated by the maximum load that can be lowered under control for three to five seconds, depending on the movement.[28] Once again, it is preferable to evaluate each leg independently.

Speed-Strength   Control tests or norms for different sports and qualification levels are itemized in tables 2.1–2.4, which may be found at the end of this chapter. Despite the paucity of such data, discretion must be used if attempting to generalize performance indices from one sport to another. For example, it may be tempting to infer that a football interior lineman's abilities should match those of a weightlifter, or that a perimeter player should match those of a sprinter. These types of assumptions, however, can lead to seriously misdirected training.

There is generally more information available on speed-strength and acceleration than on decelerative or agility parameters. Once again, however, a lesson can be taken from plyometric training.[14,28,29,36,37] The ability to decelerate from a given velocity is requisite to changing directions, just as the athlete must be able to land safely and efficiently from a given drop height before attempting depth or rebound jumps from it. An example of how to progressively evaluate this capability follows:

The athlete is instructed to achieve "second gear" (half speed) upon hearing a first whistle, and to decelerate and stop within three steps upon hearing a second whistle.

Once the athlete can satisfactorily execute this drill, a five-step braking action from "third gear" (three-quarter speed) can be introduced.

Finally, a seven-step braking action from "fourth gear" (full speed) can be implemented if appropriate.

A similar approach can be used in backward and lateral movements as well. While the choice of velocities and braking distances is somewhat arbitrary, it is imperative to establish each athlete's ability to decelerate from different speeds before attempting to redirect. As is the case with any athletic skill, this quality must be addressed progressively.

Movement Technique

Any speed, agility, and quickness training program should focus on developing the proper technique of movements that are frequently used in sports. We'll break these movements into two main categories: running mechanics and agility mechanics.

Running Mechanics   In contrast to some sport skills, running is a natural activity that most athletes have experience with (correct or otherwise). Even in the initial stages of speed, agility, and quickness training focus can often be directed toward perfecting form and correcting faults—while concurrently evaluating and developing the athlete's physical abilities—more so than toward novel mechanics. While running technique is addressed in more detail in some of the drills presented later in the book, some basic considerations will be briefly addressed here.

There are three sprinting technique variants. The drive (starting or acceleration push-off action) is emphasized during the start and acceleration, whereas the stride (full-flight striking or "pushing" action) and lift (kick-at-speed or "pulling" action) are emphasized at maximum speed.[5,8,17,22,27] The drive phase is especially important when executing speed, agility, and quickness movements. Additionally, three aspects of running mechanics are typically addressed when applying each of these technique variants:[5,8,17,22,27] eye focus (the athlete should look where he or she intends to go); arm action (the athlete should facilitate leg action with aggressive hand and knee hammering or punching motions); and leg action (the athlete should move his legs explosively and minimize ground support time). These have fundamental implications for speed, agility, and quickness movement mechanics.

Agility Mechanics   The dynamic balance, coordination, and explosiveness involved in agility movements present a unique technical challenge. For evaluative purposes, an understanding of running mechanics combined with practical experience allows some basic guidelines to be proposed.[9,10,22]

Visual Focus When Sprinting   The key role of visual focus while sprinting has important implications when executing agility drills. In general, the athlete's head should be in a neutral position and his or her eyes should be focused directly ahead regardless of whether moving forward, backward, or laterally. Exceptions to this guideline can be made when the athlete is required to focus on a teammate, opponent, projectile, or other visual target. Furthermore, directional changes (e.g., cutting left or right) and transitions (e.g., a "turn and run" maneuver from a backpedal into a forward sprint in the same direction) should be initiated by getting the head around and finding a new point of focus. Examples of coaching points that reinforce visual focus are to "open up from the top down" and "let the hips and shoulders follow the eyes." Errors may occur when the athlete initiates such actions by turning the shoulders or hips first and the eyes and head afterward, resulting in rounding off a turn or weaving outside of a desired movement path with a subsequent loss of time or efficiency.

Arm Action When Sprinting The role of arm action while sprinting—especially during the initial acceleration—also has fundamental importance when executing agility movements. The athlete must quickly accelerate into a new movement pattern and path when he is redirecting or executing transitions and turns. As is the case at the sprint start, explosive arm action should be used as a means of rapidly reacquiring high stride rate and length. Examples of coaching points that reinforce proper arm action are "punch off the line or out of the corner" (e.g., when executing the transition from a backpedal into a forward sprint in the opposite direction, or vice versa) and "punch through the turn" (e.g., during the turn-and-run maneuver mentioned above). Inadequate or improper arm action may result in a loss of speed or efficiency.

Metabolic Demands

In addition to speed-strength and technique, the metabolic demands of competition must be addressed in training and testing. The specific conditioning needed to execute technical assignments at competitive effort levels is referred to as "special endurance."[5,8,11-13,17,27,28,30,35] It is a variation on the "speed-endurance" concept that originated in racing events: the ability to maintain running speed after one to two seconds at maximal velocity, or to achieve maximum acceleration or speed during repetitive sprints. The underlying strategy is to develop the reciprocal physical and technical qualities needed to achieve a predetermined effort distribution, or a series of target paces, in competition. The training implications for sports other than race events are relatively straightforward but infrequently applied.

Competition Modeling: An Example Once a competition model has been identified, some important decisions need to be made regarding the nature and scope of tactical events to simulate in training. Consider the following analysis of the 1987 to 1991 NCAA Division I Final Four Men's Lacrosse competitions, as applied to the position of midfielder:[21,24]

- Midfield units: 3 to 4 per team
- Shifts: 9 to 14 per game (2.25 to 3.5 per quarter at 3 to 4 minute durations: 5 to 9 minute recovery)
- Continuous plays: 109.9 to 116.7 per game (5.7 to 7.5 per shift)

- Exercise/relief ratio: 30.4 to 33.2 sec : approximately 20 sec
- Proposed conditioning drill: simulate one quarter of play, each consisting of 3 midfield shifts (e.g., 8 x 150-yd shuttle run between two lines 25 yards apart):
  - 30 sec execution time
  - 20 sec relief between repetitions
  - 7 min recovery between sets

In this example, conditioning sessions are modeled on one quarter of play, during which each three-person midfield unit can expect to play approximately three shifts for three- to four-minute durations. Due to play start and stoppage patterns, shifts tend to be subdivided into six to eight repetitive exercise intervals for approximately 31.8-second durations. According to NCAA rules, play must resume within 20 seconds after each whistle (except following a goal or time out) and within 5 seconds of being signaled ready for play after a change of possession.

Both objective and subjective criteria are useful in identifying desirable segments of competition to model in training: for example, goals scored or save percentage (objective), or the coach's perception of "playing well" or "with good intensity" during certain segments of the game (subjective). Such decisions can be complicated in sports with a continuous or "transitional" character. In men's lacrosse, several other parameters (assists, ground ball retrieval percentage, scoring percentage, and shots on goal) have been shown to have useful predictive validity as well and may be helpful in making such decisions.

After assessing the type of sport you are training for, the core training or testing drills can then be selected. General examples include interval-type drills that fit the observed exercise-to-relief pattern, such as the 8 x 150-yard shuttle proposed in this example. With simple modifications, traditional "ladder" or "line" drills would be equally valid and specific. More specialized examples of possible drills include executing specific offensive, defensive, and transitional plays and tactics.

SUMMARY

The ability to rapidly decelerate, redirect, and accelerate—as well as achieve high velocities—is determined by an athlete's explosive strength. Motor skills that develop and evaluate functional speed-strength are the foundation of speed, agility, and quickness training and testing and should be implemented with respect to decelerative as well as accelerative mechanics. Reactive and explosive types of movements should be progressively introduced, in addition to basic resistance exercises and sport-specific metabolic conditioning drills.

A proper speed, agility, and quickness needs analysis involves three types of evaluation: functional strength, movement technique, and metabolic demands. As is the case with training, testing methods should dynamically correspond with the specific demands of competition, especially in regard to power and impulse application, movement patterns, and exertion level.

Test / Ranking	MALES			FEMALES		
	Average	Good	Elite	Average	Good	Elite
30 m dash	3.9 – 4.1	3.6 – 3.9	3.3 – 3.6	4.5 – 5.0	4.2 – 4.5	3.8 – 4.2
30 m (flying start)	3.5 – 3.7	3.2 – 3.5	2.8 – 3.2	4.0 – 4.4	3.7 – 4.0	3.4 – 3.7
5 double-leg bounds	13.1 – 13.7	13.7 – 14.9	14.9 – 16.7	9.2 – 11.0	11.0 – 12.8	12.8 – 15.2
5 single-leg bounds	11.3 – 12.5	12.5 – 13.7	13.7 – 15.3	10.1 – 11.3	11.3 – 12.5	12.5 – 13.7
Backward overhead weight throw	11.6 – 12.8	12.8 – 16.4	16.4 – 19.8	6.7 – 9.1	9.2 – 12.2	12.2 – 15.2

TABLE 2.1 Explosive Power Test Scores Among Male and Female College Athletes. Running times are indicated in seconds; bounding / throwing distances in meters. Data are based on a small sample of NCAA Division I-II athletes (n = 42), but provide some basis upon which to evaluate test performance.

(Adapted from Field [6])

Test / 100 m	12.8 – 13.2	12.3 – 12.7	11.8 – 12.2	11.2 – 11.7	10.7 – 11.1	10.2 – 10.6
60 m dash	6.25 – 6.65	6.55 – 6.85	6.95 – 7.35	7.35 – 7.65	7.65 – 7.95	7.95 – 8.15
30 m dash	3.65 – 3.85	3.85 – 4.15	4.1 – 4.4	4.45 – 4.65	4.6 – 5.0	5.0 – 5.1
30 m (flying start)	2.55 – 2.75	2.8 – 3.0	3.05 – 3.35	3.4 – 3.5	3.6 – 3.8	3.9 – 4.0
Long jump	2.3 – 2.6	2.4 – 2.7	2.5 – 2.8	2.6 – 2.9	2.7 – 3.0	2.9 – 3.2
Vertical jump	0.39 – 0.47	0.46 – 0.54	0.53 – 0.61	0.60 – 0.69	0.68 – 0.77	0.76 – 0.85
3 bounds	6.8 – 7.4	7.2 – 7.8	7.5 – 8.1	7.9 – 8.5	8.5 – 9.1	9.2 – 10.0
5 bounds	12.2 – 13.2	12.8 – 13.8	13.4 – 14.4	14.0 – 15.0	14.6 – 15.6	15.9 – 17.1
10 bounds	19 – 29	21 – 31	23 – 33	25 – 35	27 – 37	29.5 – 39.5

TABLE 2.2 Controls for Sprinters. Running times are indicated in seconds, jumping and bounding distances in meters. Data represent a loose guide, and given performances may be achieved without meeting all criteria.

(Adapted from Dick [5])

Test / Body Wt.	52	56	60	67.5	75	82.5	90	100	110	+110
60 m dash	7.9	7.8	7.7	7.6	7.6	7.7	7.8	7.9	7.9	8.0
5 long jumps	12	13	13.5	14	14	13.5	13.5	13.5	13.5	13
Backward overhead weight throw [7.5 kg; juniors 5.0 kg]	11	12	13	14.5	14.5	14.5	14.5	15	15	14.5
Power snatch	85 – 100	95 – 115	110 – 125	120 – 135	125 – 140	135 – 150	145 – 160	155 – 170	160 – 18-	170 – 190
Power clean	110 – 125	120 – 135	130 – 155	155 – 170	160 – 180	170 – 190	180 – 200	190 – 210	200 – 220	205 – 230
Back squat	170 – 190	180 – 200	200 – 220	210 – 230	220 – 240	230 – 250	240 – 260	260 – 280	270 – 290	275 – 300
Front squat	150 – 165	155 – 170	170 – 190	180 – 200	200 – 220	210 – 230	220 – 240	240 – 260	245 – 265	252.5 – 262.5

TABLE 2.3 Control Tests and Norms for Elite Weightlifters. Running times are indicated in seconds, jumping and throwing distances in meters, weights in kilograms.

(Adapted from Ajan and Baroga [2])

Test / Position	QB	RB	FB	TE	WR	OL	DT	DE	LB	DB
Vertical jump										
IA starters	0.72		0.80	0.75	0.79	0.66	—— 0.71 ——		0.74	0.80
IA starters		0.76			0.77	0.70	—— 0.72 ——		0.75	0.83
IA non-starters		0.74			0.73	0.63	—— 0.67 ——		0.72	0.73
IA champs '94[a]	0.81		0.79	0.76	0.81	0.67	—— 0.70 ——		0.76	0.79
IAA champs '94[a]	0.71		0.76	0.74	0.74	0.60	—— 0.74 ——		0.71	0.76
IA champs '95	0.79		0.88	0.76	0.81	0.64	—— 0.65 ——		0.78	0.82
IAA champs '95	0.76		0.84	0.91	0.86	0.66	—— 0.69 ——		0.84	0.94
IA champs '96	0.67		0.81	0.79	0.79	0.69	—— 0.79 ——		0.81	0.80
IAA champs '96	0.66		0.86	0.74	0.81	0.66	—— 0.71 ——		0.77	0.81
IA champs '97	0.78		0.80	0.75	0.94	0.62	—— 0.66 ——		0.78	0.80
IAA champs '97	0.81		0.88	0.80	0.81	0.70	—— 0.72 ——		0.81	0.85
36.6 m [40 yd] dash										
IA starters	4.79		4.57	4.76	4.57	5.13	—— 4.92 ——		4.77	4.60
IA starters		4.73			4.64	5.09	—— 4.88 ——		4.74	4.61
IA non-starters		4.79			4.81	5.16	—— 5.02 ——		4.91	4.76
IA champs '94[a,b]	4.75		4.70	5.00	4.70	5.30	—— 5.20 ——		4.95	4.70
IAA champs '94[a,b]	5.04		4.80	5.07	4.87	5.69	—— 5.10 ——		5.19	4.85
IA champs '95	4.76		4.65	4.93	4.71	5.38	—— 5.31 ——		4.91	4.73
IAA champs '95	4.80		4.60	4.90	4.60	5.05	—— 4.90 ——		4.80	4.55
IA champs '96	4.99		4.69	4.88	4.66	5.33	—— 4.69 ——		4.77	4.66
IAA champs '96	4.86		4.63	4.96	4.52	5.22	—— 4.99 ——		4.76	4.63
IA champs '97	4.73		4.78	4.97	4.75	5.36	—— 5.28 ——		4.87	4.77
IAA champs '97	4.81		4.67	4.91	4.67	5.30	—— 5.03 ——		4.76	4.59
18.3 m [20 yd] shuttle										
IA champs '95	4.12		4.07	4.27	4.14	4.55	—— 4.48 ——		4.26	4.12
IA champs '96	4.42		4.13	4.32	4.25	4.59	—— 4.46 ——		4.30	4.13
IA champs '97	4.07		4.12	4.29	4.13	4.52	—— 4.47 ——		4.20	4.11

TABLE 2.4 Positional Speed-Strength, Acceleration, and Agility Comparisons for NCAA Division I Football. Running times are indicated in seconds, jumping distances in meters. Notes: a. includes starters and other athletes with significant playing time at each position; b. measured electronically, tending to result in higher readings than those measured manually.

(Adapted from AFQ Research Staff [1], Berg, Latin, and Baechle [3], and Fry and Kraemer [7])

REFERENCES

1a. AFQ Research Staff. Champions by the numbers. *American Football Quarterly* 1(3): 88, 1995.

1b. AFQ Research Staff. Champions by the numbers. *American Football Quarterly* 2(3): 86–87, 1996.

1c. AFQ Research Staff. Champions by the numbers. *American Football Quarterly* 3(3): 85–86, 1997.

1d. AFQ Research Staff. Champions by the numbers. *American Football Quarterly* 4(3): 90–91, 1998.

2. Ajan, T., and Baroga, L. *Weightlifting: Fitness for All Sports.* Budapest: International Weightlifting Federation, Medicina Publishing House, 1988.

3. Berg, K., Latin, R.W., and Baechle, T. Physical and performance characteristics of NCAA Division I football players. *Research Quarterly for Exercise and Sport* 61(4): 395–401, 1990.

4. Delecluse, C. Influence of strength training on sprint running performance: Current findings and implications for training. *Sports Medicine* 24(3): 147–156, 1997.

5. Dick, F.W. *Sprints and Relays.* London: British Amateur Athletic Board, 1987.

6a. Field, R.W. Control tests for explosive events. *National Strength and Conditioning Association Journal* 11(6): 63–64, 1989.

6b. Field, R.W. Explosive power test scores among male and female college athletes. *National Strength and Conditioning Association Journal* 13(3): 50, 1991.

7. Fry, A.C., and Kraemer, W.J. Physical performance characteristics of American collegiate football players. *Journal of Applied Sport Science Research* 5(3): 126–138, 1991.

8. Gambetta, V., Sprints and relays. In V. Gambetta (Editor), *TAC Track and Field Coaching Manual*, 2nd Edition (pp. 55–70). TAC Development Committees. Champaign IL: Leisure Press, 1989.

9. Gambetta, V. A step in the right direction. *Training and Conditioning* 6(4): 52–55, 1996.

10. Gambetta, V. Quick to the ball. *Training and Conditioning* 7(6): 31–35, 1997.

11. Harre, D. Endurance: Classification and development. *Modern Athlete and Coach* 16(4): 19–21, 1978.

12. Harre, D. (Editor). *Principles of Sports Training.* Berlin: Sportverlag, 1982.

13. Harre, D. Facts about speed training. *Modern Athlete and Coach* 21(3): 25–27, 1983.

14. Hartmann, J., and Tunnemann, H. *Fitness and Strength Training.* Berlin: Sportverlag, 1989.

15. Hochmuth, G. *Biomechanics of Athletic Movement* (4th Edition). Berlin: Sportverlag, 1984.

16. Huijing, P.A. Elastic potentiation of muscle. In P.V. Komi (Editor), *Strength and Power in Sport* (pp. 151–168). Oxford: Blackwell Scientific Publications, 1992.

17. Jarver, J. (Editor). *Sprints and Relays: Contemporary Theory, Technique, and Training*, 3rd Edition. Los Altos, CA: Tafnews Press, 1990.

18. Komi, P.V. Neuromuscular performance: Factors influencing force and speed production. *Scandinavian Journal of Sports Science* 1(1): 2–15, 1979.

19. Komi, P.V. The musculoskeletal system. In A. Dirix, H.G. Knuttgen, and K. Tittel (Editors), *The Olympic Book of Sports Medicine* (pp. 181–193). Oxford: Blackwell Scientific Publications, 1991.

20. Komi, P.V. Stretch-shortening cycle. In P.V. Komi (Editor), *Strength and Power in Sport* (pp. 169–179). Oxford: Blackwell Scientific Publications, 1992;

21. Plisk, S.S. Regression analyses of NCAA Division I Final Four men's lacrosse competition. *Journal of Strength and Conditioning Research* 8(1): 28–42, 1994.

22. Plisk, S.S. Speed, agility, and speed-endurance development. In T.R. Baechle (Editor), *Essentials of Strength Training and Conditioning*, 2nd Edition. Champaign IL: Human Kinetics Publishers (in press), 2000.

23. Plisk S.S., and Gambetta, V. Tactical metabolic training: Part 1. *Strength and Conditioning* 19(2): 44–53, 1997.

24. Plisk, S.S., and Stenersen, S.B. The lacrosse face-off. *National Strength and Conditioning Association Journal* 14(2): 6–8 and 77–91, 1992.

25a. Schmidtbleicher, D. Strength training (part 1): Classification of methods. *Science Periodical on Research and Technology in Sport* (Physical Training/Strength W-4): 1–12, August 1985.

25b. Schmidtbleicher, D. Strength training (part 2): Structural analysis of motor strength qualities and its application to training. *Science Periodical on Research and Technology in Sport* (Physical Training/Strength W-4): 1–10, September 1985.

26. Schmidtbleicher, D. Training for power events. In P.V. Komi (Editor), *Strength and Power in Sport* (pp. 381–395). Oxford: Blackwell Scientific Publications, 1992.

27. Schmolinsky, G. (Editor). *Track and Field: The East German Textbook of Athletics*. Toronto: Sport Books Publisher, 1993.

28. Siff, M.C., and Verkhoshansky, Y.V. *Supertraining: Strength Training for Sporting Excellence*, 3rd Edition. Johannesburg: University of the Witwatersrand, 1998.

29. Soviet lecture series number 1: Depth jumps. *National Strength and Conditioning Association Journal* 9(5): 60–61, 1987.

30. Steinhofer, D. Terminology and differentiation of training methods. *Modern Athlete and Coach* 35(1): 15–21, 1997.

31. Stone, M.H. Literature review: Explosive exercises and training. *National Strength and Conditioning Association Journal* 15(3): 7–15, 1993.

32. Tidow, G. Aspects of strength training in athletics. *New Studies in Athletics* 5(1): 93–110, 1990.

33a. Verkhoshansky, Y.V. Quickness and velocity in sports movements. *New Studies in Athletics* 11(2-3): 29–37, 1996.

33b. Verkhoshansky, Y.V. Speed training for high level athletes. *New Studies in Athletics* 11(2-3): 39–49, 1996.

33c. Verkhoshansky, Y.V. Principles for a rational organization of the training process aimed at speed development. *New Studies in Athletics* 11(2-3): 155–160, 1996.

34. Verkhoshansky, Y.V., and Lazarev, V.V. Principles of planning speed and strength/speed endurance training in sports. *National Strength and Conditioning Association Journal* 11(2): 58–61, 1989.

35. Viru, A., Korge, P., and Parnat, J. Classification of training methods. *Modern Athlete and Coach* 14(5/6): 31–33, 1976.

36. Wathen, D. Literature review: Explosive / plyometric exercises. *National Strength and Conditioning Association Journal* 15(3): 17–19, 1993.

37. Zatsiorsky, V.M. *Science and Practice of Strength Training.* Champaign: Human Kinetics, 1995.

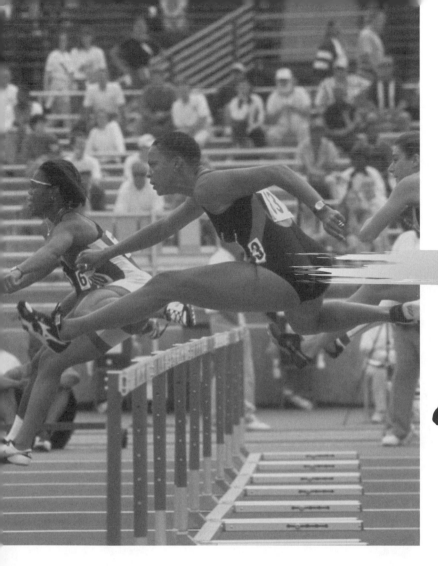

Speed Training

Doug Lentz, CSCS

Andrew Hardyk, MS

This chapter is devoted to the development of maximum running speed. This phenomenon will only last a few seconds, even for world-class athletes. Most sports outside of track sprinting do not offer the platform to showcase maximum running speed, yet sprint training does underlie the foundation of numerous sports activities. Just think of how many critical game situations in various sports are won or lost by the ability—or lack thereof—to shift into a higher gear when needed. Increasing maximum running speed has a direct correlation with increasing one's power output. The fastest runners are those athletes who spend less time on the ground, which is greatly determined by the athletes' strength and power in relation to their body composition. Although maximum speed is rarely achieved in sports, proper running mechanics and speed training will improve any athlete's sport speed.

Unfortunately, many people ascribe to the philosophy that speed is born, not made. These persons acquiesce to the notion that it is a waste of time to diligently pursue a sound speed-development program. By following the chapters in this text, there is no question that one's explosiveness, agility, acceleration, and maximum running speed can and will be improved with proper training. It is virtually impossible to discuss the topic of maximum speed without addressing the aforementioned areas as well as functional flexibility and strength or power training.

There are numerous components that make up maximum running speed outside of pure genetic potential. We will look at these important ingredients, including stride length, stride frequency, strength, power, functional flexibility, acceleration, and proper technique. In addition, this chapter will include guidelines for speed development, drills for maximum speed attainment, as well as other areas of significance that contribute to improved speed.

GUIDELINES FOR SPEED DEVELOPMENT

There is no magic formula for developing or increasing maximum running speed; however, there are some general guidelines that one should follow when training for speed improvement. Simply put, brief, intense drilling with plenty of rest between drills is critical. Sound programs will emphasize technique, starts, acceleration, speed endurance, and relaxation. The following guidelines should be adhered to:

1. All speed workouts must be performed when the body is fully recovered from previous workouts. A tired, sore, or overtrained athlete cannot improve his or her speed capabilities in a fatigued state.

2. Proper sprinting technique must be taught and mastered by the athletes. To master skills they must be performed correctly through many repetitions to reinforce the skill acquisition.

3. All sets and repetitions of a speed workout must be followed by adequate rest. The athlete's heart rate and respiration should return to almost normal levels after the drill. Any sprint drill that lasts six to eight seconds, at maximum or near maximum effort, will have implications on the ATP-PC, and more importantly the CNS. Both of these very important systems need almost full recovery to make maximal efforts possible. A 1:4-6 work-to-rest ratio is recommended as a general rule.

4. Speed workouts should be varied between light, medium, and heavy days. For example, back-to-back hard days would not be beneficial to speed enhancement.

5. Track the total distance run by the athletes during each maximum speed workout.

6. To achieve one's maximum speed, the athlete must learn to run in a relaxed mode. This is much easier said than done, especially with junior and senior high non-track athletes.

7. Speed endurance can be accomplished by running longer intervals (150 meters to 400 meters) or by decreasing the rest between short intervals (10 to 20 meters). For most sports applications, repeating shorter intervals is more applicable and specific.

ACCELERATION

For most sports, acceleration, which is the rate of change of velocity, is the most important component of speed development and attainment. Following the start, all athletes will accelerate by increasing both stride length and stride frequency.

One way to increase stride length and stride frequency is to increase overall functional strength through the entire body. Improved strength levels will allow athletes to produce greater amounts of force while at the same time decreasing their ground contact time. Training the body to use the attained strength gains in a powerful fashion is the key to acceleration improvement. Power refers to the ability to generate the greatest amount of force (strength) in the shortest possible time. In a nutshell, the most powerful athletes spend less time on the ground, have longer strides, and can repeat them more rapidly than their less powerful counterparts.

The highest rates of acceleration are achieved in the first 8 to 10 strides taken by an athlete. Close to 75 percent of maximum running velocity is established within the first 10 meters. Maximum running speed will be reached within four to five seconds. As mentioned earlier, true maximum running speed will seldom be attained in most sporting situations outside of track sprinting.

To ensure a proper transition to top speed, quick running steps should increase in length gradually until full stride length is achieved. Explosive starting actions require application of concentric forces through the hip, knee, and ankle joints, and the execution of the quick running steps requires tremendous elastic strength in the hip, knee, and ankle musculature. Good hip-joint mobility will assist athletes with leg separation during the "knee-lift phase." Elastic or eccentric strength should prevent the leg from collapsing in the knee, hip, and ankle regions during impact with the ground. This elastic strength also reduces the time that the foot is in contact with the ground (amortization phase).

SPORT-SPECIFIC SPEED

The speed used in sports rarely allows 100 percent of maximum speed to be used. In most cases, quick bursts of speed are required to catch a ball or overtake an opponent. These short bursts of speed that are specific to the individual activity are what are referred to as "sport speed." In essence, sport-specific speed is a blend of agility, acceleration, and speed.

Stride Frequency

Stride frequency is defined as the number of strides taken in a given amount of time or distance. By improving stride frequency, the athlete will be able to decrease the time between his or her strides while at the same time maintaining or even increasing stride length. This will result in increased overall speed. Good technique is fundamental to increasing stride frequency.

Sprint-assisted training is one technique that can also be used to improve stride frequency. Assisted sprinting will allow the athletes to develop the feel of running at a faster velocity than they would be capable of running normally. This added dimension of supramaximal speed will enable the athletes to improve their running mechanics at a faster pace than would be possible unassisted. By not having to run at 100 percent capacity, but still being able to achieve a speed that is at or slightly above their unassisted best, the athletes can learn to relax at high speed more easily.

Some of the traditional assisted methods of training include downhill running and towing. All athletes should be well versed in the mechanics of proper sprinting form before attempting this type of training. All downhill running sessions must be preceded by a proper warm-up and stretching routine, followed by low- to medium-intensity acceleration sprints. For athletes new to this type of training, it might be beneficial to begin with low-intensity sprints on a flat surface.

Stride Length

Stride length is the distance covered in one stride during running. Research has found that optimal stride length at absolute speed is related to the athlete's leg length (normally 2.3 to 2.5 times the athlete's leg length). A common mistake of many young athletes is to try to take steps that are too long in an effort to attain top speed. When this happens, athletes have a tendency to overstride and ultimately slow themselves down. Most athletes will develop their optimal stride length as proper technique, strength, and power improve.

Stride length can be developed by improving the athletes' elastic strength. Elastic strength is the ability to quickly transition from eccentric to concentric muscle actions, especially during the plant phase of running. There are numerous modalities used to improve elastic strength, including resistance training, plyometrics and resisted running, weighted vests, running chutes, and harnessed and uphill running. Coaches must be careful not to get too carried away with the different forms of "resisted methods" of training. One of the potential negative effects of overutilized resisted running training could be a decrease in mechanical effeciency. There does not appear to be one single mode of resisted running training that is superior to the others. A coach's decision to try these devices will be based on the training level of the athlete, economics, time available to train the athletes, space allotment, and familiarity with the aforementioned modes of training.

PROPER SPRINT MECHANICS

Sprint mechanics is another term for sprint form or sprint technique. Proper mechanics allow the athlete to maximize the forces that the muscles are generating so that the highest speed predicted by the athlete's genetic potential and training can be achieved. Good technique also increases neuromuscular efficiency which, in turn, allows smooth coordinated movements that will facilitate faster running speed.

There are three main elements to concentrate on regarding proper sprinting mechanics: posture, arm action, and leg action. Posture refers to the alignment of the body. The athlete's posture changes depending on the phase of the sprinting action. During acceleration, there is more of a pronounced lean ($\sim$45 degrees) that aids in overcoming inertia. As the athlete approaches his or her maximum running speed, the posture should become more erect ($\sim$70 degrees). Regardless of the phase of sprinting, one should be able to draw a straight line from the ankle of the supporting leg through the knee and the hip, then another straight line through the torso and head (see figures 1 and 2). Arm action refers to the range of motion and velocity with which the athlete uses the arms. Vigorous and coordinated arm movement is necessary in all phases of sprinting, but in the initial acceleration phase it is critical. The arm swing counteracts leg and hip rotational forces (e.g., right leg and left arm). This counterbalance allows the body to stay aligned in the intended direction. Asynchronous arm action will detract from one's maximum running speed. Leg action is the relationship of the hips and legs relative to the torso and ground. Explosive starts require extending the hip, knee, and ankle to produce the greatest force possible against the ground.

PROPER SPRINTING POSITION

"Proper sprinting position" refers to the body's posture during sprinting movements. There are several requirements to keep in mind when coaching speed mechanics:

1. Head position: The head should be in line with the torso and the torso should be in line with the legs at all times. Do not allow the head to sway in any direction. Try to maintain a relaxed upright position with the jaw relaxed and loose.

2. Body lean: Body lean does not come from any one body part. Running can be seen as a controlled fall. The body should have a slight forward lean during acceleration. At maximum speed the torso should be erect and tall. Have the athletes concentrate on complete extension of the hip and knee joint as the foot pulls the hips over and complete knee pickup of the recovery leg.

3. Leg action: The foot should be maintained in a dorsiflexed (toes up) position throughout the running cycle except when the foot is in contact with the ground. At this point the weight should be on the ball of the foot (never on the heel) directly under the athlete. As the foot leaves the ground, it follows a path straight up toward the buttocks. Simultaneously, the knee raises up and the thigh is almost parallel to the ground. The foot then drops down below the knee. At this point the knee is at an angle of approximately 90 degrees. The leg straightens down and underneath the body. This process is repeated with the other leg. The greater the running speed, the higher the heel should kick up. Failure to achieve a high rear heel kick will slow the speed of the leg turnover rate. Avoid placing the front foot too far in front of the center of gravity. Practice running as lightly as possible with correct foot-ground contact.

4. Arm action: Aggressive arm action is a must. Each arm should move as one piece with the elbow bent at about 90 degrees. Hands remain relaxed, and should come up to about nose level in the front and should pass the buttocks in the back. Arm action is always straight forward and backward, never side to side. Arm swing should originate from the shoulder and not involve excessive flexion and extension of the arms.

As top speed is approached:

- The head must be held high.
- The torso becomes more upright.
- The shoulders and head are relaxed.
- The driving leg should be fully extended to the ground.

Adhering to the drills listed at the end of this chapter will ensure proper technique and thus improved running speed.

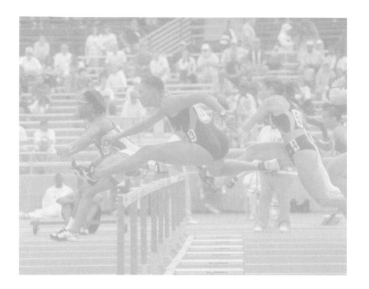

Drills for Speed Development

Although sport speed rarely involves 100 percent top-end speed, top-end speed work can be utilized for various purposes.

Some of the drills require a "quick release" system of attachment. Belts are recommended over harness attachments due to their closer location to the body's center of mass and reduced interference with upper body and postural running mechanics. The use of Velcro belts allows an athlete to quickly remove a resistance device and transition into a nonassisted environment. In essence, the neuromuscular system sees this alleviated condition as an acute and short-lived "over-speed" condition.

The most common error in assisted or resisted "speed" work is providing too much assistance or resistance. Although several authors provide different guidelines, a good general rule is to provide no more than 10 percent assistance (i.e., 10 percent reduction in time for any given distance) or resistance (i.e., 10 percent increase in time for any given distance). You may apply this general rule to all resisted and assisted "speed" drills.

- Maximum speed mechanics prevail over speeds of about 70 to 80 percent of maximum speed.

- Proper execution of top-end speed drills teaches and emphasizes proper locomotive mechanics.

- Maximum speed mechanics allow the athlete to participate in a variety of drills that will reinforce proper locomotive mechanics as well as provide excellent multidimensional athletic development.

- Proper locomotive skills allow more versatility in the conditioning program.

Since sport speed contains a large accelerative component, "pure" acceleration drills have been included in this section.

These speed drills will target maximum speed mechanics. A high position start is used to start the drill, with a 5- to 10-yard buildup. This eliminates the acceleration component of locomotion. After the athlete has mastered the basic locomotive mechanics of maximum speed and acceleration, integrating acceleration and speed drills provides a more comprehensive and functional approach to sport speed development. Resisted and assisted runs are included in drills 41 through 47.

Standing Stationary Arm Swings

Arm Action Drills

PURPOSE

Improve running mechanics and speed by providing teaching cues to the upper body while in a stationary position

PROCEDURE

- Stand with feet together and swing arms in a sprinting motion.

- Each arm should move as one piece with the elbow bent at about 90 degrees.

- Keep hands relaxed.

- Hands should come up to about shoulder level in the front and should pass the gluteus in the back.

- The arm action should be forward and back without crossing the main line of the body.

VARIATIONS

- Seated Arm Swings—The athlete is seated on the floor with the legs straight out in front. Be careful not to bounce off of the floor as the drill becomes more vigorous. This drill will help train the correct position of the arms as the hands pass the lowest point of the swing by avoiding contact with the ground.

- Weighted Arm Swings—Use light dumbbells in the hands to work on shoulder strength. Use enough resistance to provide a good training stimulus but not enough to alter good arm mechanics.

- Contrast Resisted Arm Swings—Perform arm swings with 1- to 2-pound weights for 10-20 arm swings, then drop the weights and perform 10-20 arm swings without resistance.

Note: This section will focus on pure locomotive acceleration. The quickness chapter will focus on transitional acceleration, involving body position changes. Unless otherwise indicated, perform the drills over a 10- to 20-yard distance.

2

Running Balance

Basic Technique Speed Drills

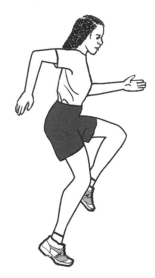

PURPOSE

Increase muscle stiffness at ankle complex

PROCEDURE

- Get into the "foot plant" position of maximum speed: posture upright; arms at 90 degrees with the left hand at shoulder level and the right hand at hip level; right knee up with the right heel close to gluteus; left leg slightly bent and only the ball of left foot making ground contact.

- Hold the position for 20-60 seconds.

- Make the drill more demanding by using a weight vest or belt, or standing on an unstable surface (e.g., foam pad or mat).

COMPLEX VARIATION

- Assume a one-leg balance in a sport-specific position (e.g., kicking in karate)

- Add motion to free leg or upper body (e.g., kicking while standing on one leg)

Ankling

Basic Technique Speed Drills

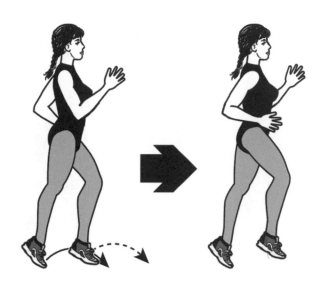

PURPOSE

Increase foot speed and elastic ankle strength

PROCEDURE

- Jog with very short steps, emphasizing the plantar flexion phase of ground contact and low foot recovery. Keep quiet but fast feet. Land and push off the ball of the foot. Minimize ground contact and maximize foot contacts.

4

Straight Leg Shuffle

Basic Technique Speed Drills

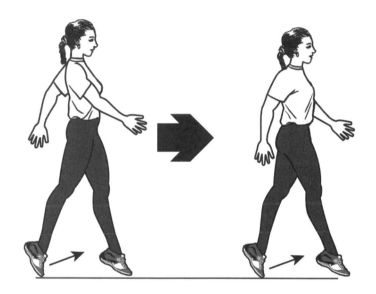

PURPOSE

Increase hip strength and elastic ankle strength

PROCEDURE

- Run keeping the legs straight and the foot dorsiflexed.
- Emphasize fast ground contact with the ball of the foot and pulling through with the hips.

Butt-Kickers

Basic Technique Speed Drills

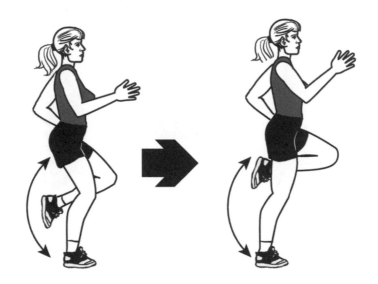

PURPOSE

Increase foot speed

PROCEDURE

- From a jog, pull the heel of the lower leg up to and bounce off the gluteus.

- As the leg bends, the knee should come forward and up.

6

Wall Slides

Basic Technique Speed Drills

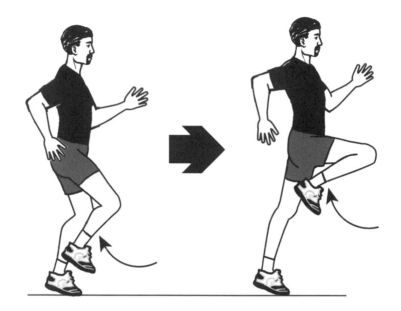

PURPOSE

Improve knee lift and enhance frequency of turnover

PROCEDURE

- Same as Butt-Kickers, but do not allow the heel of the recovery leg to travel behind the body.

Paw Drill (Cycling)

Basic Technique Speed Drills

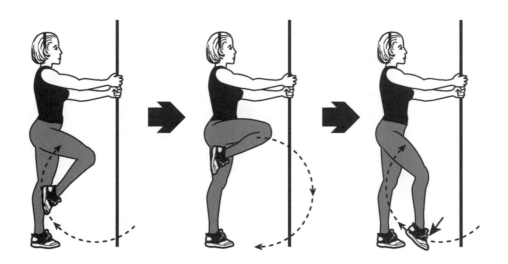

PURPOSE

Increase frequency of turnover

PROCEDURE

- Using a supporting structure for balance, cycle one leg in a sprinting manner.

- Try not to let the recovering foot cycle behind the body.

- Allow the foot to kick the gluteus during the recovery, pawing the ground to finish the action.

8

"A" March Walk

Supplemental Speed Drills

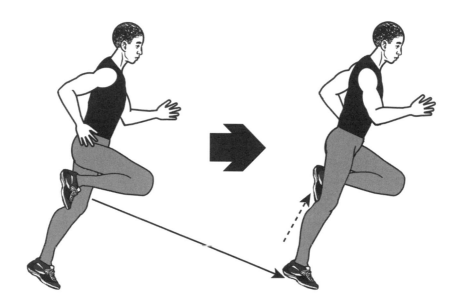

PURPOSE

Increase foot speed

PROCEDURE

- March using perfect posture and arm action.
- The knee on the recovery leg should be brought high, while staying fully flexed, keeping the ankle close to the gluteus and dorsiflexed.
- When the recovery knee is at the highest point, the opposite "ground" foot should emphasize plantar flexion.

"A" Skips

Supplemental Speed Drills

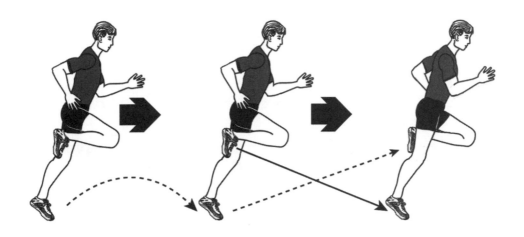

PURPOSE
Increase hip extension, flexion strength, and ankle muscle stiffness

PROCEDURE
- Skip with the same mechanics discussed in the "A" March Walk.
- While in the air, emphasize the high recovery posture used in the "A" March Walk.
- Keep the upper body in an upright and steady position at all times.
- The foot strike should be quiet but explosive, emphasizing muscle stiffness at ankle.
- Be careful not to slam the foot onto the ground.

COMPLEX VARIATION
- "A" Form Runs—Perform form runs emphasizing the pronounced mechanics practiced in the "A" Skips.

10

Single-Leg Fast Legs

Supplemental Speed Drills

PURPOSE

Increase turnover and enhance leg recovery speed

PROCEDURE

- Jog with a very low foot recovery with one leg and perform an "A" motion with the other leg.

- This pattern can be changed to every other step, or to a predetermined number of steps, or be performed on command.

- The high-knee "A" motion is always performed with the same leg.

VARIATION

- Alternating Fast Legs—Same as Single-Leg Fast Legs, except alternate the "A" motion between the right and left legs.

"B" March

Supplemental Speed Drills

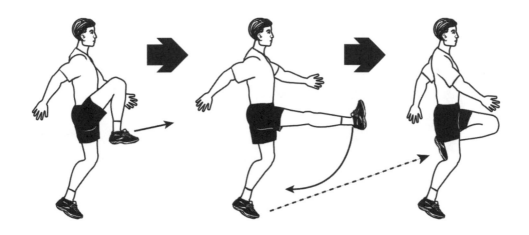

PURPOSE

Improve hip extension mechanics and enhance hamstring firing

PROCEDURE

- March as you did in the "A" March Walk.
- Allow the recovering leg to extend in front of you after a high-knee block.
- Paw down and dive the hips through.

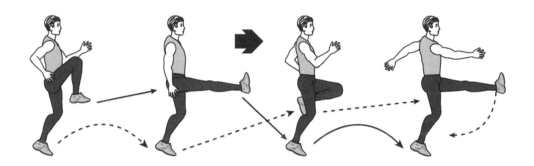

12

"B" Skips

Supplemental Speed Drills

Purpose

Increase stride length and frequency as well as enhance hamstring and hip performance

Improve muscle stiffness at the ankle complex

PROCEDURE

- Perform the "B" leg movement (i.e., the recovery leg's knee blocks high as possible), while skipping.

- Emphasize a quick leg extension followed by an explosive hip extension (pawing) and drive the hips through.

COMPLEX VARIATION

- "B" Form Runs—Run while using the "B" series leg movements.

Resisted Stationary "A" Skips

Supplemental Speed Drills

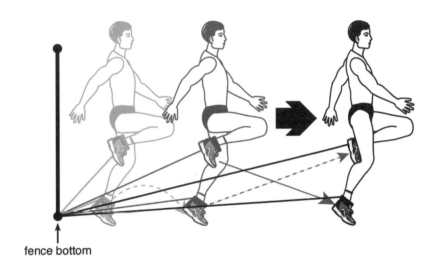

fence bottom

PURPOSE

Improve stride frequency and strengthen hip flexion, as well as en-hance heel recovery mechanics

PROCEDURE

- Attach a 5- to 7-foot rubber (surgical) tubing to each of your ankles.
- Secure both tubings to the bottom of a fence or post.
- Face away from the fence and step away about 6 to 8 feet.
- Perform stationary "A" Skips.

14

Speed

Resisted Stationary "B" Skips

Supplemental Speed Drills

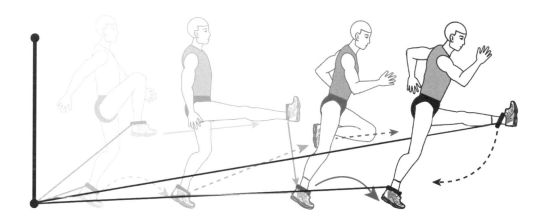

PURPOSE

Increase stride length and frequency as well as enhance hamstring and hip performance

Improve muscle stiffness at the ankle complex

PROCEDURE

- Attach a 5- to 7-foot rubber (surgical) tubing to each of your ankles.

- Secure both tubings to the bottom of a fence or post.

- Face away from the fence and step away about 6 to 8 feet.

- Perform stationary "B" Skips.

Ladder Speed Run

Agility Ladder (Stick) Drills

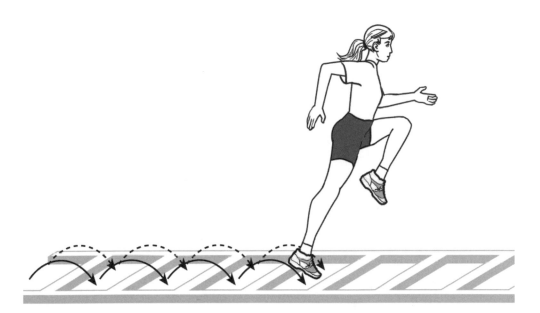

PURPOSE

Enhance timing and stride frequency while teaching quick turnover

PROCEDURE

- Run through an agility ladder (i.e., sticks 18 inches apart) as fast as possible, touching one foot down between each rung.

- Emphasize high knee lift and quick ground contact.

16

Ladder Stride Runs

Agility Ladder (Stick) Drills

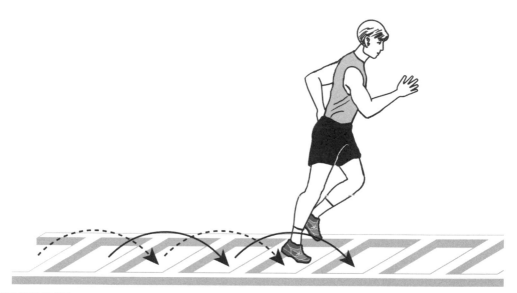

PURPOSE

Enhance timing and stride frequency while teaching quick turnover

PROCEDURE

- Run through an agility ladder (i.e., sticks 18 inches apart) as fast as possible, touching one foot down between every other rung.

- Emphasize upright posture with sound arm and leg mechanics.

Single-Leg Run Through

Hurdle Drills

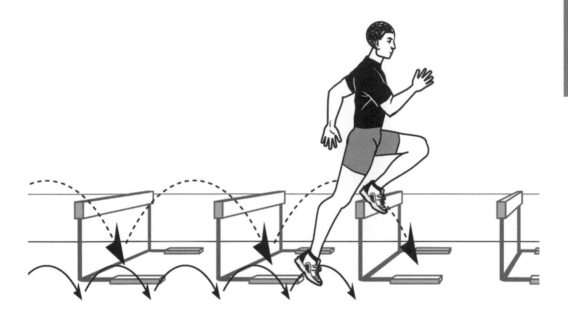

PURPOSE

Enhance stride frequency while strengthening hip flexors and improving lower-body ambidexterity

PROCEDURE

- Set 8 to 10 6- to 12-inch hurdles about 3 feet apart.

- Run with one leg outside the hurdles and the other going over the hurdles.

- Emphasize a straight outside leg (as in a shuffle) and a quick "A" motion on the "hurdling leg" (e.g., as in an "A" motion).

Run Through

Hurdle Drills

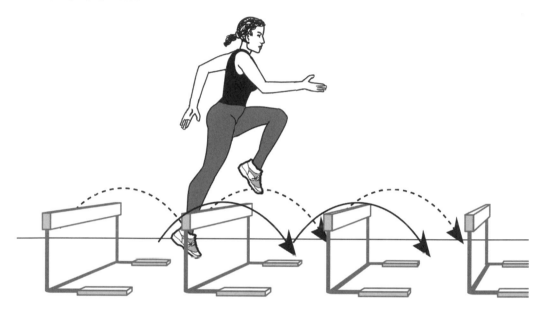

PURPOSE

Enhance stride frequency while strengthening hip flexors and improving lower-body ambidexterity

PROCEDURE

- Set 8-10 6- to 12-inch hurdles about 3 feet apart.

- Perform an "A" run over the hurdles.

- Emphasize quick "knee up/toe up" with a quick heel-to-gluteus recovery.

- Perform the exercise with a two-foot strike between each hurdle (maintaining the same lead leg through the drill), or faster with a one-foot strike between hurdles.

Hurdle Fast Legs

Hurdle Drills

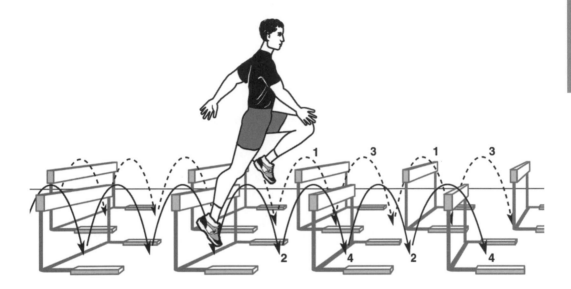

PURPOSE

Enhance stride frequency while strengthening hip flexors and improving lower-body ambidexterity

PROCEDURE

- Stagger 8 to 10 6- to 12-inch hurdles so that half line up with the right leg and the other half line up with the left leg.

- The hurdle pattern should be a hurdle for the left leg, followed by a hurdle 3 feet apart for the right leg; repeat pattern.

- The leg sequence is the left foot over the left hurdle, then two steps in between the hurdles.

20

"Against the Wind" Speed Runs

Resisted Speed Drills

PURPOSE

Increase stride length and running strength

PROCEDURE

- Run against a steady wind using perfect maximum speed running mechanics.

Light Sled/Tire Pulls

Resisted Speed Drills

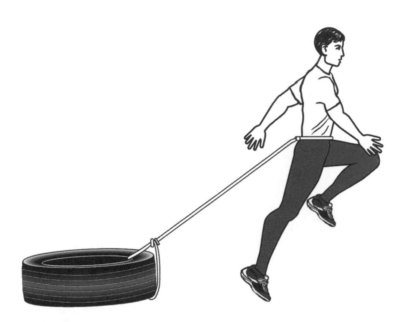

PURPOSE

Enhance running strength and power and improve stride length

PROCEDURE

- Attach athlete to a weighted sled or car tire, which the athlete then drags behind.

- Emphasize proper sprinting mechanics.

- Do not make the sled so heavy that acceleration mechanics are needed to pull it.

22

Uphill Speed Runs (1- to 3-Degree Incline)

Resisted Speed Drills

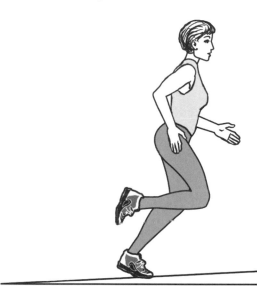

(1- 3° for running speed

PURPOSE

Enhance running strength and power and improve stride length

PROCEDURE

- Gravity provides resistance on uphill runs. Emphasize perfect maximum speed mechanics.

- Do not exceed a 3-degree incline if the goal is to develop maximum running speed.

- Higher inclines are more appropriate for acceleration mechanics and will be discussed in that section of this chapter.

Partner Tubing-Resisted Speed Runs

Resisted Speed Drills

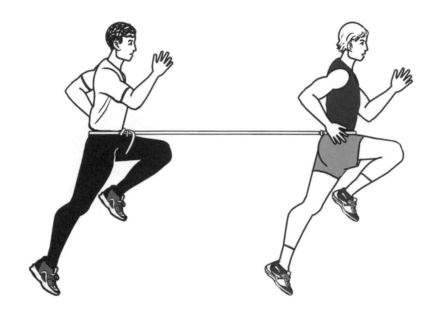

PURPOSE

Enhance running strength and power and improve stride length

PROCEDURE

- Attach two athletes at the waist with a 10- to 20-yard rubber tubing.

- They line up at a distance 2 to 5 yards longer than the cord.

- They begin running at the same time.

- The rear athlete tries to maintain the same distance to provide constant resistance to the front athlete.

24

Parachute Running

Resisted Speed Drills

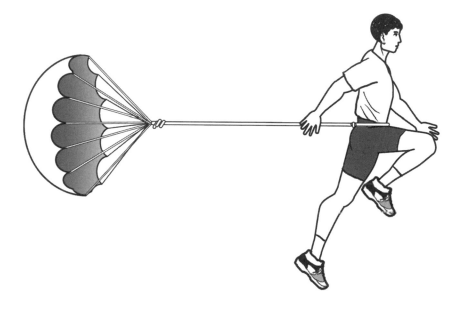

PURPOSE

Enhance running strength and power and improve stride length

PROCEDURE

- Athlete wears a belt with a small parachute attached by a cord.
- Parachute deploys with 0 to 4 steps (depending on wind conditions and parachute model) and provides extra air resistance.

Sand Running

Resisted Speed Drills

PURPOSE

Increase stride length and hip strength

PROCEDURE

- Sprinting on the beach in loose sand makes sprinting more difficult and can provide good resistance training. It also provides increased proprioception to the locomotive environment.

26

Contrast Parachute Running

Contrast Resisted Runs

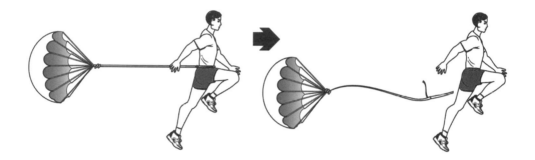

PURPOSE

Enhance stride length of start and turnover at top speed
Increase starting speed and transition to top speed

PROCEDURE

- The athlete attaches a parachute, which is dragged behind during the run.

- Emphasize proper speed mechanics.

- After a buildup and 10 to 20 yards of near maximum running, release the Velcro belt to allow unresisted running.

- The athlete should feel an "over speed" sensation over the next 10 to 20 yards.

Uphill-to-Flat Contrast Speed Runs (5-Degree Incline)

Contrast Resisted Runs

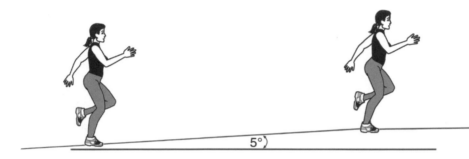

5°

PURPOSE

Enhance stride length of start and turnover at top speed
Increase starting speed and transition to top speed

PROCEDURE

- Position yourself 10 to 20 yards below the top of the hill (15- to 20-degree hill).

- Quickly build up to near maximum speed by the time you are 10 to 15 yards below the top of the hill.

- Continue to increase speed as you go over the hill to flat ground.

- Hit a higher gear as you transition to the flat ground, running an additional 15 to 25 yards over the flat ground.

28

Contrast Sled/Tire Pulls

Contrast Resisted Runs

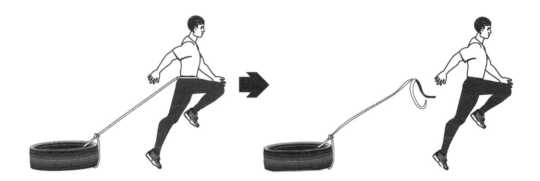

PURPOSE

Enhance stride length of start and turnover at top speed
Increase starting speed and transition to top speed

PROCEDURE

- Attach a weighted-sled or car tire to the athlete, which the athlete will drag behind during the run.

- Emphasize proper speed mechanics.

- After a build up and 10 to 20 yards of near maximum running, re-lease the Velcro belt to allow unresisted running.

- The athlete should feel an "over speed" sensation over the next 10 to 20 yards.

"With the Wind" Speed Runs

Assisted Speed Drills

PURPOSE

Increase top end speed and stride frequency

PROCEDURE

- Run with a steady wind at your back using perfect maximum speed running mechanics.

30

Partner Tubing-Assisted Speed Runs

Assisted Speed Drills

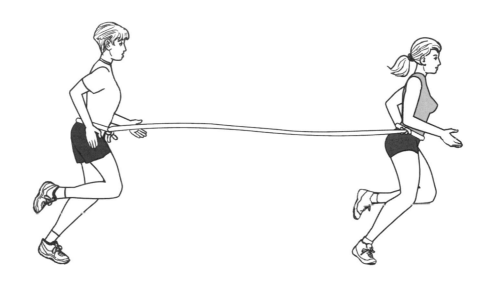

PURPOSE

Increase top end speed and stride frequency

PROCEDURE

- Two athletes are attached at the waist by a 10- to 20-yard rubber tubing.

- They line up at a distance 2 to 5 yards longer than the cord.

- They begin running at the same time.

- The front athlete tries to maintain the same distance to provide constant assistance to the rear athlete.

- Runs should be 20 to 40 yards in length.

Downhill Speed Runs (3- to 7-Degree Decline)

Assisted Speed Drills

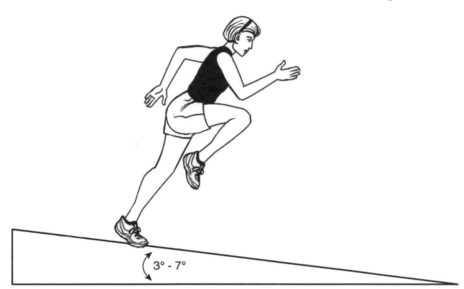

3° - 7°

PURPOSE

Increase top end speed and stride frequency

PROCEDURE

- Gravity provides assistance on downhill runs.

- Emphasize perfect maximum-speed mechanics.

- Do exceed a 3- to 7-degree decline if the goal is to develop maximum running speed, but overstriding will result in deceleration and interfere with speed development.

- A grass surface is preferred over asphalt due to safety concerns involving falls.

Partner Tubing-Assisted to Unassisted Speed Runs

Contrast Assisted Runs

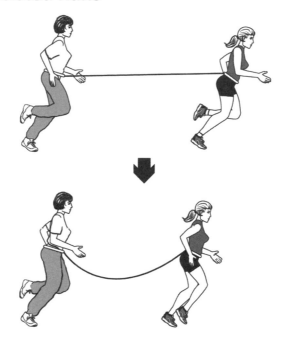

PURPOSE

Increase top end speed and stride frequency

PROCEDURE

- Two athletes are attached at the waist by a 10- to 20-yard rubber tubing.

- They line up at a distance 2 to 5 yards longer than the cord.

- They begin running at the same time.

- The front athlete tries to maintain the same distance for 10 to 20 yards to provide constant assistance to the rear athlete.

- The front athlete then slows down slightly to allow the rear athlete to run unassisted for 10 to 20 additional yards.

- Run should be 20 to 40 yards in length.

Downhill-to-Flat Contrast Speed Runs (3- to 5-Degree Decline)

Contrast Assisted Runs

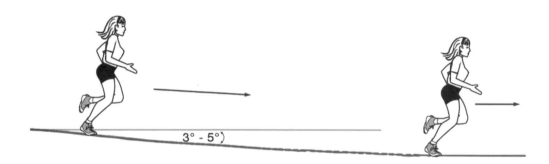

3° - 5°)

PURPOSE

Increase top end speed and stride frequency

PROCEDURE

- Position yourself 10 to 20 yards above the bottom of the hill.
- Quickly build up to near maximum speed by the time you are about 5 yards above the bottom of the hill.
- Continue to increase speed as you transition to flat ground.
- Try to maintain "supramaximal speed" through the transition and on to the flat ground, running for an additional 10 to 15 yards.

Note: The objective of these drills is to try to maintain "supramaximal" speed for 2-3 seconds in the absence of assistance.

34

Wall Drills (Acceleration Marches)

Basic Technique Acceleration Drills

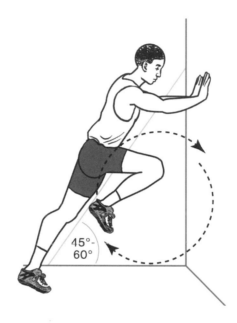

45°-
60°

PURPOSE

Enhance muscle stiffness at ankle complex and improve elastic strength of the lower body

PROCEDURE

- Lean against a wall at about a 45- to 60-degree angle with your arms supporting the body.
- Stay on the balls of the feet at all times.
- Bring one knee up, simulating the acceleration position.
- From this position, bring the recovery leg down and the plant leg up.
- You can perform any number of cycles of this procedure (e.g., 1, 3, 5, or for time).

Falling Starts

Basic Technique Acceleration Drills

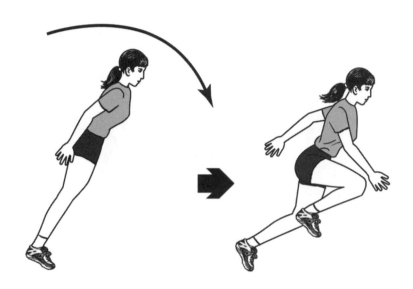

PURPOSE

Enhance quick leg turnover at start and teach the proper acceleration lean

PROCEDURE

- Athlete stands with feet together and leans forward until balance is lost.

- Athlete then accelerates at full speed to catch him- or herself.

- Athlete runs 20 to 30 yards.

36

Moye (Crouched Variation) Starts

Basic Technique Acceleration Drills

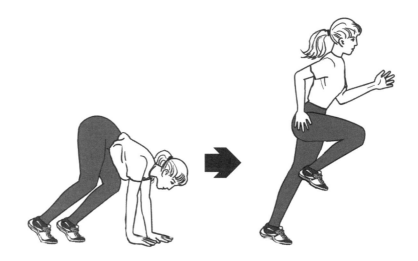

PURPOSE

Improve reaction time and starting response and enhance first step quickness and acceleration mechanics

PROCEDURE

- Moye starts provide several positions from which to start from, including standing, three-point, and four-point starts.

- For a three- or four-point start, assume the desired position with the hands placed on the ground about two foot lengths in front of the front foot.

- Begin to lean forward and "explode" when the shoulders go beyond the hands.

Basic 40-Yard Model

Basic Technique Acceleration Drills

PURPOSE

Teach starting, acceleration, and maximum speed integration
Enhance 40-yard test performance

PROCEDURE

- For 40-yard sprint times greater than 4.7 seconds, follow this sequence: visualize the start, inhale, assume starting position, hold your breath, and GO; then split arms, drive back leg, push-push (focus on hard leg drives) for about 10 yards, exhale and inhale, drive tall in an upright posture, and at about 20 yards exhale and inhale, step over knees, and finish tall.

- For 40-yard sprint times less than 4.7 seconds, follow this sequence: visualize, inhale, assume starting position, hold your breath, and GO; then split arms, drive back leg, push-push about 15 yards, exhale and inhale, drive tall, step over knees, and finish tall.

38

Gears

Supplemental Acceleration Drills

PURPOSE

Improve transition acceleration and enhance ability to change speeds (gears)

PROCEDURE

- Space 5 cones 20 yards apart.

- Varying running intensity between cones will teach you to accelerate and shift (transition) between various speeds (i.e., gears).

- For example, run in second gear between cones 1 and 2, third gear between cones 2 and 3, first gear between cones 3 and 4, and fourth gear between cones 4 and 5.

- You can change the order of the gears to any order you wish.

- You can also use fewer cones for specific transition work or more cones for conditioning work.

Ins (15 Yards) and Outs (15 Yards)

Supplemental Acceleration Drills

PURPOSE

Improve transition acceleration and enhance ability to change speeds (gears)

PROCEDURE

- Space 5 cones 15 to 30 yards apart.

- Start at first cone.

- Accelerate to submaximum speed by the second cone.

- At the third cone, try to go faster than you have ever have attempted to go (try to break your maximum speed record).

- At cone four, reduce intensity but try to maintain frequency.

40

Acceleration Runs (17-Inch and 4-Inch)

Acceleration Ladder (Stick) Drills

PURPOSE

Enhance acceleration and top end running by teaching proper striding

Prevent deceleration due to overstriding

PROCEDURE

- A special ladder is placed on the running surface (sticks may also be used).

- Set up the acceleration ladder rungs, or the 18-inch-long sticks, in the following sequence: 17 inches between rungs 1 and 2; add 4 inches to next distance, for 21 inches between rungs 2 and 3; add 4 inches to next distance, for 25 inches between rungs 3 and 4; and so on.

- Each rung is placed 4 inches farther apart than the previous distance between rungs up to the maximum desired stride length of the athlete.

- As the athlete accelerates, he or she is paced by the rungs.

- This drill promotes proper foot placement and prevents "overstriding."

41

Weighted Starts

Resisted Acceleration Drills

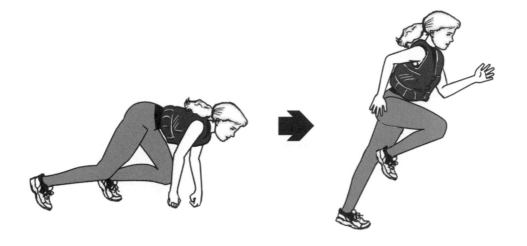

PURPOSE

Enhance elastic strength of start

PROCEDURE

- Using a weighted vest, or shot belt, will enhance the neural reflex of any start.

Note: This section will focus on pure locomotive acceleration. The quickness chapter will focus on transitional acceleration, involving body position changes. Unless otherwise indicated, perform drills 41 through 54 over a 10- to 20-yard distance.

42

Stadium Stairs

Resisted Acceleration Drills

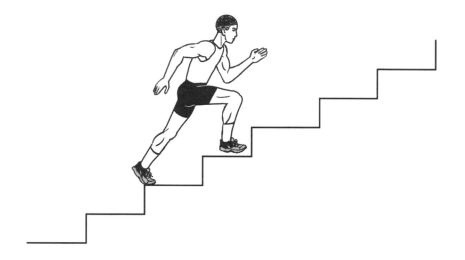

PURPOSE

Enhance starting power and stride length

PROCEDURE

- Run up stadium stairs or bleachers for 4 to 8 seconds.

Uphill Acceleration Run

Resisted Acceleration Drills

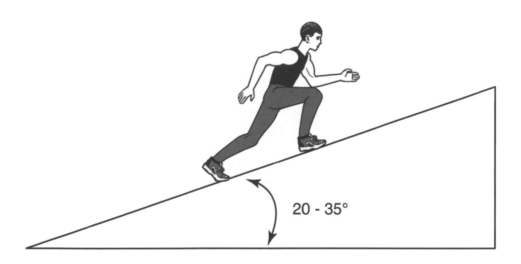

20 - 35°

PURPOSE

Enhance starting power and improve stride length during acceleration

PROCEDURE

- Use a 20- to 35-degree hill.
- Take 4- to 8-second runs up the hill.
- Count your strides and mark your spot at your chosen time.
- Try to beat the distance with fewer strides in subsequent timed runs.

eavy Sled Pulls

tion Drills

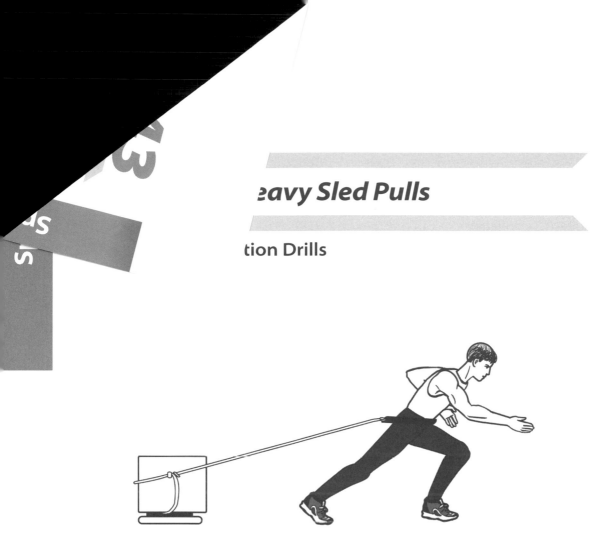

PURPOSE

Enhance starting power and stride length

PROCEDURE

- Attach a weighted sled to the athlete, which the athlete then drags behind during a 15- to 20-yard acceleration run.

- Explosive starts and acceleration mechanics are emphasized.

45

Partner-Resisted Starts

Resisted Acceleration Drills

Speed

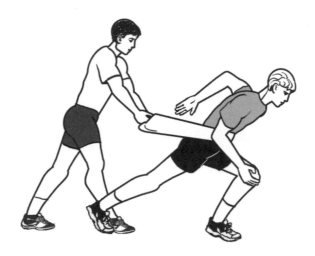

PURPOSE

Enhance starting power and stride length

PROCEDURE

- An athlete can be resisted during the first 8 to 10 strides by a partner.
- The resisting partner is situated in front of the running partner with the hands on the shoulders; or the resisting partner works from the back, using hands or a towel around the waist of the running partner to resist the start and acceleration phase.
- The drill ends after 8 to 10 strides.

Speed

Partner Tubing-Assisted Acceleration Drill

Assisted Acceleration Drills

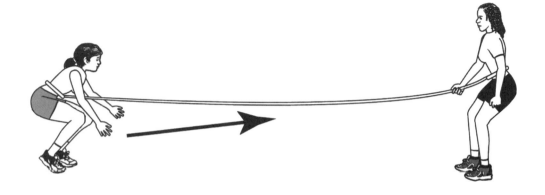

PURPOSE

Improve quick leg recovery at first few steps
Enhance stride frequency during acceleration

PROCEDURE

- Two athletes are attached at the waist by a 10- to 20-yard rubber tubing.

- The "assisting" athlete lines up at a distance 15 to 25 yards from the "assisted" athlete.

- The "assisted" athlete gets into the ready position of choice and explodes at the GO signal for 10 to 20 yards with the aid of the rubber tubing.

- For longer acceleration runs, the "assisting" athlete can run at the GO signal to provide continued assistance for a longer duration.

Towed Running (Pulley)

Assisted Acceleration Drills

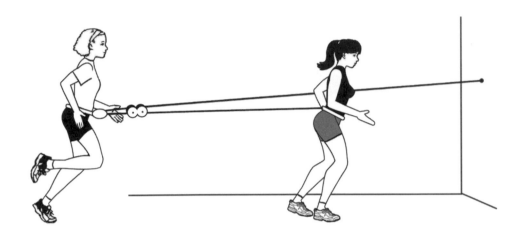

PURPOSE

Increase acceleration

PROCEDURE

- Two athletes are connected by a rope and pulley system that allows one athlete to be towed while the other athlete runs at half the speed of the towed athlete.

- The towed athlete runs faster than under normal conditions.

Speed

Partner-Assisted Let-Go's

Contrast Acceleration Drills

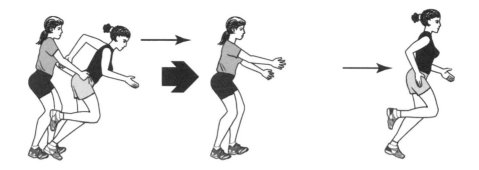

PURPOSE

Teach quick transitions in speed and enhance stride frequency of acceleration

PROCEDURE

- Have a partner use his or her hands, a towel, or rope to hold you at about a 45-degree forward lean.

- Start running, pumping the legs and arms explosively.

- Have the partner let you go after about 5 strides.

- Feel yourself explode out of the falling position, using fast leg and arm movements to recover from the falling sensation.

Bullet Belt

Contrast Acceleration Drills

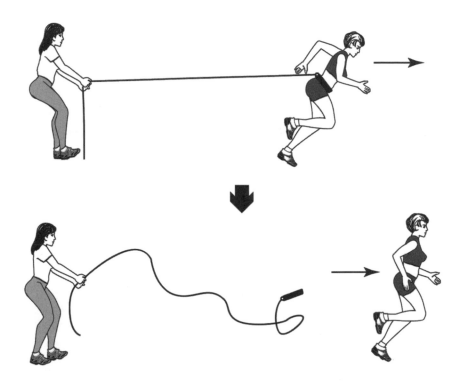

PURPOSE

Teach quick transitions in speed and enhance stride frequency of acceleration

PROCEDURE

- The bullet belt allows an athlete to be held (i.e., by a partner) while he or she is attempting to accelerate until enough force is applied that the Velcro strip holding the running athlete breaks.

- There are several techniques used to release the accelerating athlete, including the rip and the pop methods.

50

Skip for Height

Plyometric Drills

PURPOSE

Increase hip extension and flexion strength and ankle muscle stiffness

Improve leg power and enhance stride length

PROCEDURE

- Skip, driving the free knee upward as aggressively as possible.
- Make the arm action very aggressive as well.
- Try to skip as high as possible on each jump.

51

Skip for Distance

Plyometric Drills

PURPOSE

Increase hip power and stride length

PROCEDURE

- Skip, driving the knee upward and forward as aggressively as possible.
- Make arm action equally as aggressive.
- Try to skip as high as possible.

Split-Squat Jumps

Plyometric Drills

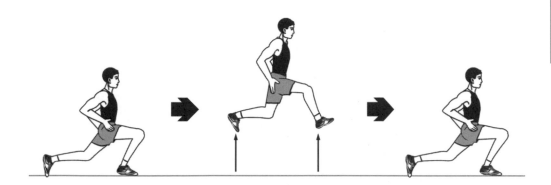

PURPOSE

Increase hip power and stride length

PROCEDURE

- Start in a lunge position.
- Jump straight into the air and return to the original position.
- Repeat without pausing.
- The knee closest to the ground should never touch the ground.
- The hands are placed on the hips, or may be used in unison to drive upward with each jump.
- Repeat for the other leg.

VARIATION

- Alternating Split-Squat Jumps—On each jump the legs switch positions and the other leg is in front at ground contact.

Bounding

Plyometric Drills

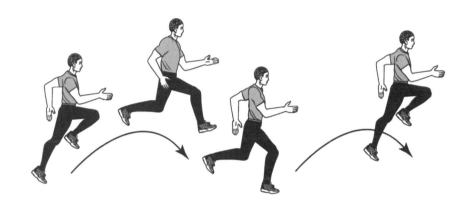

PURPOSE

Increase hip extension and flexion strength and ankle muscle stiffness

Improve leg power and enhance stride length

PROCEDURE

- Run, but drive the free knee so that the thigh reaches a parallel position with the ground and jump a little on each step.

- This should look like a bouncy run with longer than normal strides.

- Be careful not to reach forward at ground contact.

Single-Leg Bounds

Plyometric Drills

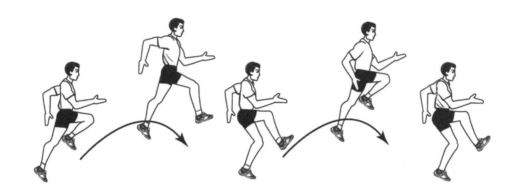

PURPOSE

Increase hip extension and flexion strength and ankle muscle stiffness

Improve leg power and enhance stride length

PROCEDURE

- Get a slow running start and start hopping on a single leg.

- You can measure improvement by checking the distance in a given number of hops.

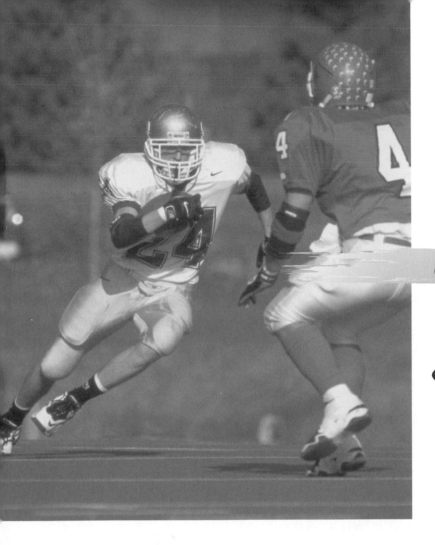

Agility Training

John F. Graham, BS, CSCS

Sports rarely are performed straight ahead, but rather require changes of direction in which lateral movements are used in the several planes of movement simultaneously. Be it the World Cup or Wimbledon, the ability to move side to side and up and down rapidly is essential to championship athletic performance.

Most sports are played in short bursts of 30 feet or less before a new course of action is needed. And because these movements are initiated from various body positions, athletes must be strong, explosive, and quick from every possible postural alignment.

Agility is defined as the ability to decelerate, accelerate, and change direction quickly while maintaining good body control without decreasing speed.[1,3,4,7,8] Agility is closely related to balance because it requires athletes to regulate shifts in the body's center of gravity while subjecting them to postural deviation.[3]

Athletes who develop their multidirectional quickness are more likely to excel. Whether it is a basketball player cutting toward a pass or a football lineman pulling to make a trap block on a defensive lineman, agility is a critical and often overlooked component of athletic performance.[1] In sports such as baseball, lateral speed, agility, and quickness can be just as essential to success as strength and speed.[7]

Improvements in agility are directly correlated to enhanced athletic timing, rhythm, and movement.[4] Little wonder then that today's scouts, coaches, and players place such a high premium on this athletic attribute. Great agility isn't just a bonus for volleyball, soccer, and other team sport players who must move swiftly on their feet, it's a requirement.

AGILITY TRAINING BENEFITS

While enhanced athletic performance is an overriding aim, dedicated agility can provide additional rewards. Even athletes who will never make spectacular Michael Jordan-like moves benefit from agility work.

A primary effect of agility training is increased body control resulting from a concentrated form of kinesthetic awareness. This form of training appears to help athletes control small adjustments in neck, shoulder, back, hip, knee, and ankle joints for the optimal postural alignment during performance.

Moreover, agility training gives athletes a greater sense of control in making fast movements. Athletes in a variety of sports report excellent gains in athleticism through effective, frequent agility workouts. This seems to be especially true for less coordinated athletes, who demonstrate and feel a greater increase in control as a result of their training than do more coordinated peers.[8]

While injuries will never be eliminated from sports, proper overall conditioning combined with functional agility training can help reduce their occurrence. Athletes with greater agility are often able to control the potential injury-causing mechanism as it begins. By controlling the body at that split-second—the critical instant of impact, twist, or turn—an injury can often be avoided or reduced in its severity. Athletes can't be prepared for every awkward movement or collision, but by imitating multidirectional sports movements under low to moderate stress levels in practice, they can develop a neuromuscular awareness that triggers the injury-preventive response in certain situations.

The rehabilitation process can also be speeded by a highly developed neuromuscular awareness. Athletes with such awareness can better read their bodies as they respond to treatment than can athletes who have less developed kinesthetic sense.

To review, the potential payoffs of agility training include increased

- power, balance, speed, and contraction;
- intramuscular coordination;
- explosiveness of the major muscle groups;
- quickness;
- ability to repeat high-intensity work; and
- coordination of skills.

Fortunately, once developed, agility declines less quickly than does speed, strength, or endurance. Agility training leaves a more lasting mark upon muscle memory. In athletic terms, an agility workout is like putting money in the bank.

AGILITY DRILLS FOR MAXIMUM RESULTS

The key to improving agility is to minimize loss of speed when shifting the body's center of gravity. Drills that require rapid changes of direction forward, backward, vertically, and laterally help improve agility as well as coordination by training the body to make those changes in movement more quickly.[3,7] Over the past three decades, sports conditioning programs have incorporated more dynamic drills that maximize the development of high-performance physical tools, including agility.

Agility drills can be divided into three categories. In programmable agility drills the athlete knows beforehand what the movement combinations will be. In reactive agility drills the athlete is required to respond instantly to the movement of another athlete or to the signals of a coach. In quickness drills the athlete is required to perform fast foot movements as quickly as possible.

Programmable, reactive, and quickness agility drills come in many forms. The number of movements and apparatuses that can be incorporated include line, backpedal, bag, jump rope, rope, agility ladder, cone, plyometric box, slide board, and sidekick box drills.

For the greatest benefit, agility drills should be implemented as most appropriate for the training cycle and sport, from both a metabolic and performance-enhancement perspective. Workouts should progress at a proper level with regard to speed, distance, and volume. Strength training and other forms of conditioning should augment agility work in adequate proportions in a periodized program.

The goal of a quality agility training program is to make adaptations as needed. Shifts from one mesocycle to another (hypertrophy > strength > power > competition > transitional) offer opportune times to adjust the level and type of agility work being performed. Agility drill selection should be based on the physiological and biomechanical needs of the athlete at that point in time, the available resources, and the training environment to ensure safe and effective training sessions. Keep these variables in mind as you design and implement your agility program.

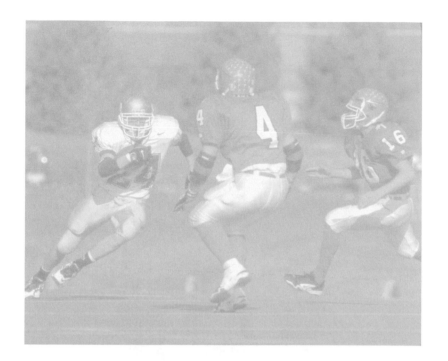

Drills for Agility Development

Due to the obvious overlap between some of the drills in this book, this agility section will concentrate on transitional movements. Although we include changes of direction, we will also emphasize fluid changes in body positions and level changes.

55

Carioca

Assorted Biomotor Skills

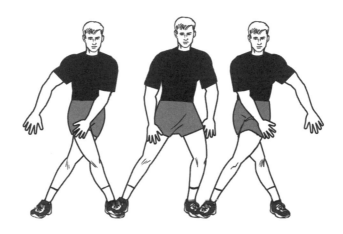

PURPOSE

Development of balance, flexibility in hips, footwork, and lateral speed

PROCEDURE

- Start in a two-point stance.
- Begin standing sideways at one end of the ladder.
- Laterally step with the right foot over the left leg.
- Cross the left foot behind the right leg.
- Step with the right foot in front of the left leg.

COMPLEX VARIATION

- Tapioca—Just like the Carioca, but with smaller and faster steps.

Agility

Crossover Skipping

Assorted Biomotor Skills

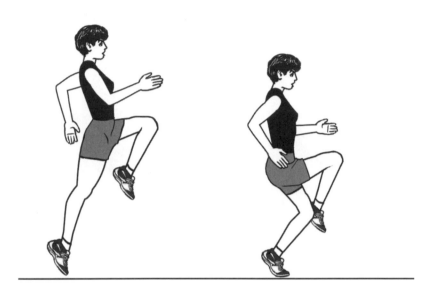

Agility

PURPOSE

Develop explosive cross-over mechanics for direction changes
Develop explosive contralateral hip flexon and extension

PROCEDURE

- Start in a two-point stance.

- Begin skipping laterally to your left crossing the right leg over the left.

- Emphasize left hip extension and right hip flexion.

- Rotate the hips to the left as the right leg goes over and in front of the left.

- Keep shoulder square to the front.

20-Yard Shuttle (Pro Agility)

Line Drills

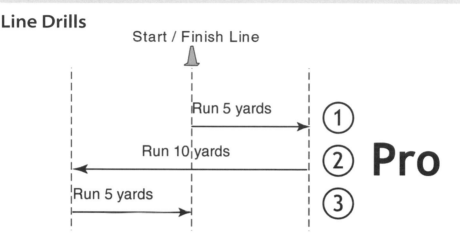

PURPOSE

Development of change of direction, footwork, and reaction time

PROCEDURE

- Start in a two-point stance straddling the starting line.
- Turn to the right, sprint, and touch a line 5 yards away with your right hand.
- Turn back to the left, sprint 10 yards, and touch the far line with your left hand.
- Turn back to the right, sprint 5 yards through the start line to the finish.

COMPLEX VARIATION

- 20-Yard Combination Agility Drill—Perform different biomotor skills on each leg of the line drill.

Note: There are an infinite number of permutations of line drills. By changing the distance and order of the drill a new variation can be created. Level changes can also be added to all line drills to add complexity. For example, a squat thrust, or push-up, can be added at every cone.

T-Drill

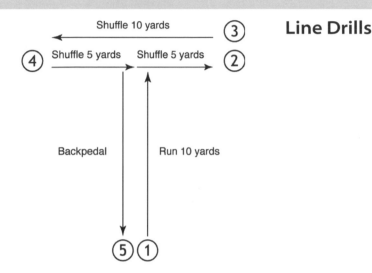

Shuffle 10 yards

③

Line Drills

④ Shuffle 5 yards   Shuffle 5 yards ②

Backpedal   Run 10 yards

⑤①

PURPOSE

Development of agility, conditioning, flexibility in abductors and adductors, and transition between the three major skills (run, shuffle, and backpedal)

PROCEDURE

- Start in a two-point stance.
- Sprint forward 10 yards to a marked spot on the ground.
- Side shuffle to the right and touch a line 5 yards away with your right hand.
- Shuffle back to the left for 10 yards and touch the far line with your left hand.
- Shuffle back to the right for 5 yards to the marked spot.
- Touch the marked spot with either foot and backpedal 10 yards through the start line to the finish.

COMPLEX VARIATION

- Make the cones any distance that mimics the "sport distance" you are working on.
- Vary the biomotor skill during each leg of the drill.

59

Squirm

Line Drills

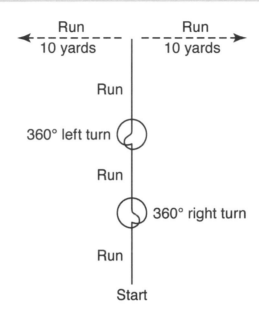

Run ← 10 yards — — — Run 10 yards →

Run

360° left turn

Run

360° right turn

Run

Start

Agility

PURPOSE

Development of footwork and reaction time

PROCEDURE

- Start in a two-point stance.
- Sprint forward 5 yards.
- Rotate 360 degrees, and sprint another 5 yards.
- Rotate 360 degrees, and sprint another 5 yards.
- Sprint right or left for 10 yards.

COMPLEX VARIATION

- Put your right hand down on the ground during the first right 360 and your left hand down on the ground during the second 360.
- Vary the distance.
- Make turns on command by coach.
- Use various biomotor skill combinations throughout the drill.

40-Yard Ladder Sprint

Line Drills

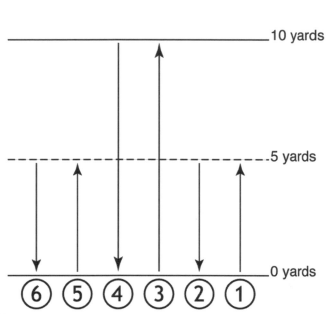

Agility

PURPOSE

Development of agility and conditioning

PROCEDURE

- Start in a two-point stance on the starting line.

- Sprint 5 yards to the first line, touch the line with your right hand, return to the starting line, and touch it with your left hand.

- Sprint 10 yards to the second line, touch the line with your right hand, return to the starting line, and touch it with your left hand.

- Sprint 5 yards to the first line, touch the line with your right hand, and return to the starting line.

COMPLEX VARIATION

- Combine biomotor skills during each leg of drill.

- Start the drill from various positions (e.g., lying, sitting, etc.).

- Add tumbling to each turn.

61

15-Yard Turn Drill

Cone Drills

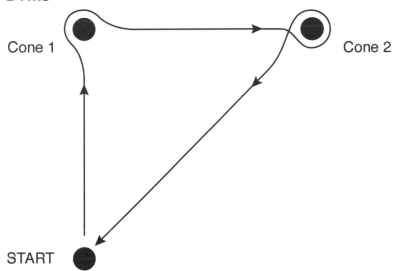

PURPOSE

Change of direction, flexibility in hips, and footwork

PROCEDURE

- Start in a two-point stance.
- Sprint forward 5 yards to the first cone, and make a sharp right turn around it.
- Sprint to the second cone (located 5 yards to the right of the start and diagonal from the first cone), and make a left turn around the cone.
- Sprint 5 yards through the finish.

COMPLEX VARIATIONS

- Put inside hand on the ground when making turns.
- Change cone distance.
- Make turns on command, not at cones.

20-Yard Square

Cone Drills

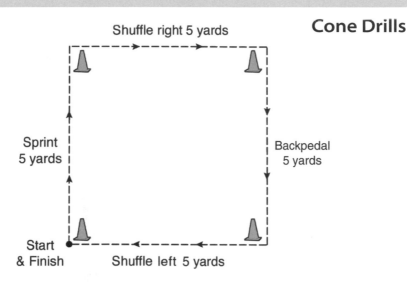

Shuffle right 5 yards

Sprint 5 yards

Backpedal 5 yards

Start & Finish

Shuffle left 5 yards

PURPOSE

Improve change of direction and body position, transitions between skills, and cutting ability

PROCEDURE

- Start in a two-point stance
- Sprint 5 yards to first cone, make sharp right cut.
- Shuffle right 5 yards, make a sharp cut back.
- Backpedal 5 yards to next cone, make sharp left cut.
- Left shuffle through finish.

COMPLEX VARIATION

- Start from different positions (e.g., lying, four-point stance, etc.).
- Change distance of cones to appropriate distance for sport and energy system.
- Change skills of each leg to meet specific needs.
- Cut with inside or outside leg.
- Cut on the outside of the cone or circle around the cones.
- Put inside hand on the ground during turns.

63

X-Pattern Multi-Skill

Cone Drills

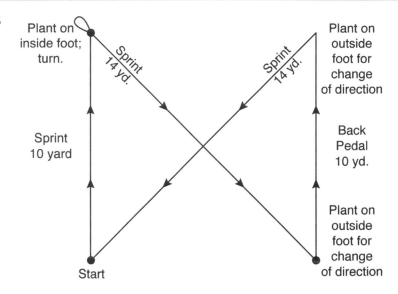

Plant on inside foot; turn.

Plant on outside foot for change of direction

Sprint 14 yd.

Sprint 14 yd.

Sprint 10 yard

Back Pedal 10 yd.

Plant on outside foot for change of direction

Start

Agility

PURPOSE

Improve transitional movement and cutting ability

PROCEDURE

- Start in a two-point stance.
- Sprint 10 yards to the first cone.
- At the first cone sprint diagonally 14 yards to the second cone.
- Backpedal 10 yards to the third cone.
- At the third cone, sprint diagonally 14 yards to the fourth cone.

COMPLEX VARIATION

- Start from different positions (e.g., lying, four-point stance, etc.).
- Change distance of cones to appropriate distance for sport and energy system.
- Change skills of each leg to meet specific needs.
- Cut with inside or outside leg.
- Cut on the outside of the cone or circle around the cones.
- Put inside hand on the ground during turns.

Figure Eights

Cone Drills

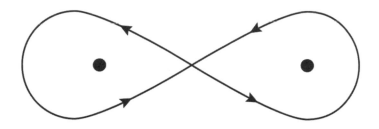

Agility

PURPOSE

Change of direction and reaction development

PROCEDURE

- Position two flat cones 5 to 10 yards apart.

- Start in a two-point stance.

- Run a figure eight between the cones, placing your inside hand on the cone while you make the turn.

COMPLEX VARIATION

- Change the distance between cones.

- Change the radius of the turns.

- Start drill from various positions (e.g., lying, sitting, four-point stance, etc.).

65

Z-Pattern Run

Cone Drills

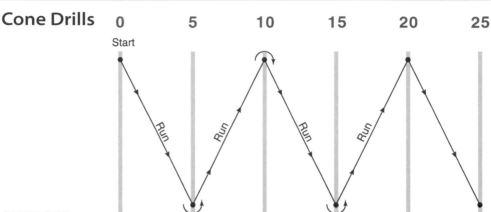

PURPOSE

Improve transitional movement and turning ability

PROCEDURE

- Position three cones on two lines 5 yards apart such that the cones on line 1 are at 0, 10, and 20 yards, and the cones on line 2 are at 5, 15, and 25 yards.
- Start in a two-point stance.
- Sprint diagonally 5 yards to the first cone, plant the outside foot and run around the cone.
- Continue to sprint diagonally to each cone, running around each cone.

COMPLEX VARIATION

- Start from different positions (e.g., lying, four-point stance, etc.).
- Change distance of cones to appropriate distance for sport and energy system.
- Change skills of each leg to meet specific needs.
- Cut with inside or outside leg.
- Cut on the outside of the cone or circle around the cones.
- Put inside hand on the ground during turns.

Agility

Zigzag

Cone Drills

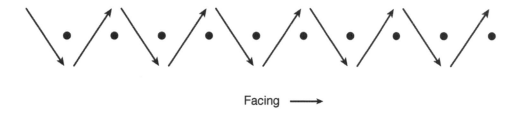

Facing ⟶

PURPOSE

Footwork and change of direction skills

PROCEDURE

- Start in a two-point stance.
- Stand facing a row of 10 cones, each cone 1 yard apart.
- Step forward quickly and diagonally with the right foot to the right of the first cone, and then slide the left foot to the right foot.
- Lead with the left foot to the left side of the next cone, and then slide the right foot to the left foot.
- Zigzag through all the cones quickly and explosively.

COMPLEX VARIATION

- Start from different positions (e.g., lying, four-point stance, etc.).
- Change distance of cones to appropriate distance for sport and energy system.
- Change skills of each leg to meet specific needs.
- Cut with inside or outside leg.
- Cut on the outside of the cone or circle around the cones.
- Put inside hand on the ground during turns.

67

Z-Pattern Cuts

Cone Drills

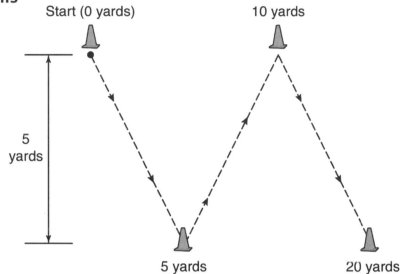

Start (0 yards) 10 yards

5 yards

5 yards 20 yards

PURPOSE

Improve cutting ability

PROCEDURE

- Place cones as indicated above.

- Start in a two-point stance.

- Sprint to first cone, plant on outside leg and cut sharply towards the next cone.

COMPLEX VARIATION

- Start from different positions (e.g., lying, four-point stance, etc.).

- Change distance of cones to appropriate distance for sport and energy system.

- Change skills of each leg to meet specific needs.

- Cut with inside or outside leg.

- Cut on the outside of the cone or circle around the cones.

- Put inside hand on the ground during turns.

Icky Shuffle

Agility Ladder Drills

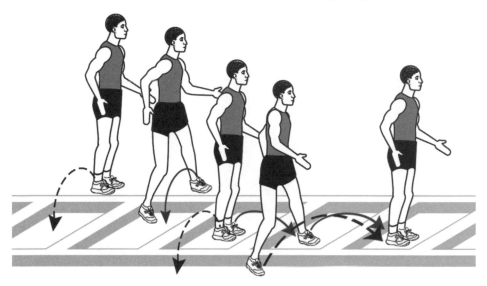

Agility

PURPOSE

Enhance coordination and improve lower-body quickness

PROCEDURE

- Start on the lefft side of the ladder.

- Lateral step with the right foot and place it in the first square, then the left foot follows the right foot inside the first square of the ladder.

- Lateral step with the right foot to the right side of the ladder, then advance the left foot to the next square in the ladder.

- Bring the right foot to the square the left foot is in.

- Lateral step to the left side of the ladder and advance the right foot to the next square on the latter.

- Repeat pattern.

Note: To add complexity to all ladder drills, look up during the drill and avoid looking at your feet. Perform all drills forward and backwards.

69

Carioca

Agility Ladder Drills

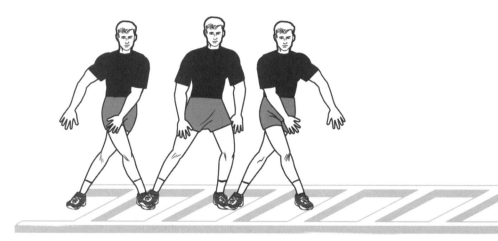

PURPOSE

    Development of balance, flexibility in hips, footwork development, and peripheral vision

PROCEDURE

- Start in a two-point stance.
- Begin standing sideways at one end of the ladder.
- Cross-step with the right foot into the first square in front of the left leg.
- Cross the left foot into the second square. The left foot should cross behind the right leg.
- Cross-step with the right foot into the third square. The right foot should cross behind the left foot.
- The left foot crosses over in front of the right foot into the next square.
- Repeat this sequence through the ladder.
- Emphasize a fast hip rotation with fast foot placement.

In-Out Shuffle

Agility Ladder Drills

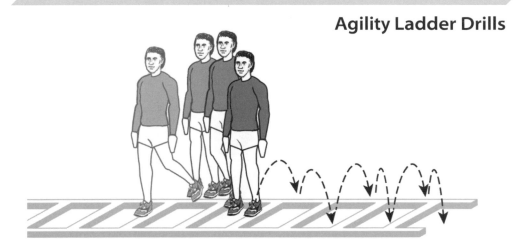

Agility

PURPOSE

Agility, balance, coordination, and quickness development

PROCEDURE

- Start in a two-point stance.
- Begin standing sideways to the ladder, with the ladder in front of you.
- Step with the left foot straight-ahead into the first square.
- Follow with the right foot into the first square.
- Step back and diagonally with the left foot until it is in front of the second square.
- Follow with the right foot until it is in front of the second square.
- Repeat this sequence throughout the ladder.
- Each foot hits every box.

COMPLEX VARIATION

- Perform same pattern with each foot in a separate box.
- Use every other box and increase lateral step.
- Perform backwards (i.e., start with the ladder behind you).

71

Side Right-In

Agility Ladder Drills

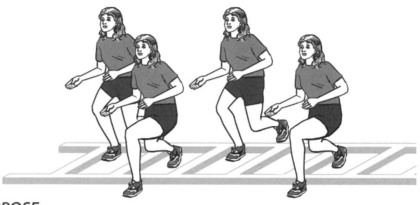

PURPOSE

Agility, balance, coordination, and quickness development

PROCEDURE

- Start in a two-point stance.
- Begin standing sideways to the ladder with the ladder in front of you.
- Step with the right foot into the first square.
- Step forward with the left foot over the first square to the other side of the ladder.
- Step laterally with the right foot to the second square.
- Step backward with the left foot over the ladder until it is in front of the second square.
- Step laterally with the right foot to the third square.
- Repeat this sequence throughout the ladder.
- Remember: the right foot is always in, but the left foot is never in.

COMPLEX VARIATION

- Increase lateral step and use every other box.

Side Left-In

Agility Ladder Drills

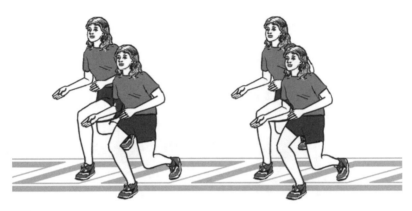

Agility

PURPOSE

Agility, balance, coordination, and quickness development

PROCEDURE

- Start in a two-point stance.
- Begin standing sideways to the ladder with the ladder in front of you.
- Step with the left foot into the first square.
- Step forward with the right foot over the first square to the other side of the ladder.
- Step laterally with the left foot to the second square.
- Step backward with the right foot over the ladder until it is in front of the second square.
- Step laterally with the left foot to the third square.
- Repeat this sequence throughout the ladder.
- Remember: the left foot is always in, but the right foot is never in.

COMPLEX VARIATION

- Increase lateral step and use every other box.

73

Crossover Shuffle

Agility Ladder Drills

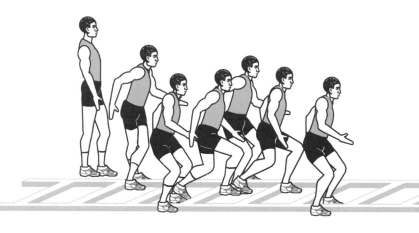

PURPOSE

Increase flexibility and power in the hips
Improve change of direction

PROCEDURE

- Stand with ladder to your right.
- Cross over with left foot to the first square of the ladder.
- Laterally step with the right foot to the right side of the ladder.
- Immediately cross over with the right foot to the second square of the ladder.
- Laterally step with the left foot to the left side of the ladder.
- Repeat.
- Remember: only one foot is in the ladder at any one time.

Zigzag

Agility Ladder Drills

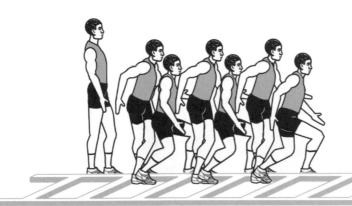

Agility

PURPOSE

Increase crossover mechanics
Improve rotational capabilities

PROCEDURE

- Stand with the ladder to your right.

- Cross over with your left to the first square of the ladder.

- Step your right foot behind and over your left foot so it lands on the left side of the ladder.

- Step your left foot behind and over your right foot so it lands on the second square of the ladder.

- Repeat.

- Remember: left foot is always in the ladder and the right foot is always outside the ladder.

COMPLEX VARIATION

- Perform the zig zag across the ladder, with no foot contact inside the ladder.

75

Zigzag Crossover Shuffle

Agility Ladder Drills

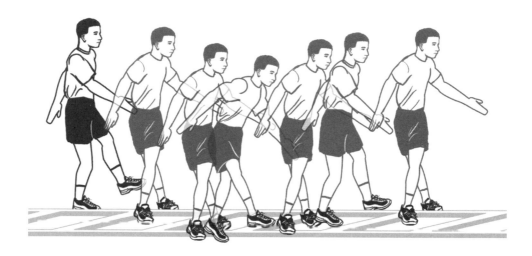

PURPOSE

Flexibility in abductors and adductors, foot coordination, and change of direction

PROCEDURE

- Start in a two-point stance.
- Starting at the left side of the agility ladder, perform a crossover step with the left foot in front of the right foot into the first square.
- Bring the right leg behind the left leg to the right side of the first square.
- Laterally step with the left leg to slightly outside the right side of the first square.

- Crossover with the right leg in front of the left leg to inside the second square.
- Bring the left leg behind the right leg to the left side of the second square.
- Laterally step with the right leg to slightly outside the left side of the second square.
- Continue down the agility ladder in this pattern.

VARIATION
- Perform drill backwards.
- Start in a two-point stance on the left side of the ladder facing backwards.
- Perform a crossover step with the right foot in front of the left foot into the first square.
- Bring the left leg behind the right leg to the right side of the first square.
- Laterally step with the right leg in front of the left leg to slightly outside the right side of the first square.
- Crossover with the left leg behind the right leg to inside the second square.
- Bring the right leg in front of left leg to the left side of the second square.
- Laterally step with the left leg to slightly outside the left side.
- Continue down the agility ladder in this pattern.

76

Snake Jump

Agility Ladder Drills

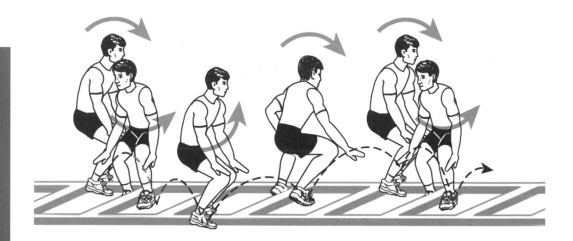

PURPOSE

Development of agility, balance, coordination, hip flexibility, and quickness

PROCEDURE

- Start in a two-point stance, straddling one side of the ladder.
- Keeping both feet together perform a series of quarter-turn jumps.
- The direction the feet should point for each jump is as follows: straight-ahead, right, straight-ahead, left, straight-ahead, and so on.
- This drill forces you to rotate the hips with each jump.

180-Degree Turn

Agility Ladder Drills

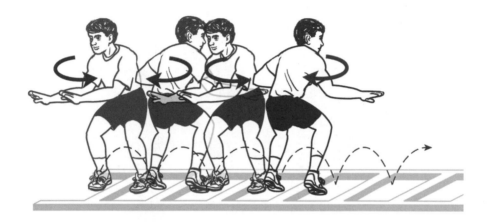

Agility

PURPOSE

Agility, balance, hip flexibility, and quickness development

PROCEDURE

- Start in a two-point stance, straddling the first rung of the ladder.
- With both feet jump and turn 180 degrees, and land straddling the next rung.
- Continue repeating the half turns into every square through the agility ladder.

VARIATION

- Drill can be performed facing perpendicular to the ladder.

78

Slalom Ski Jump

Agility Ladder Drills

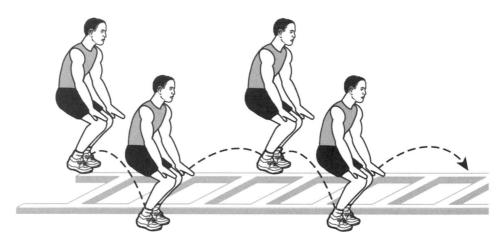

Agility

PURPOSE

   Agility, balance, coordination, and quickness development

PROCEDURE

- Start in a two-point stance.

- Begin at one end of the agility ladder.

- Keeping both feet together, jump back and forth over of the ladder in a zigzag pattern.

- This drill may also be performed on one leg, as you become more experienced.

COMPLEX VARIATION

- Perform while jumping backwards.

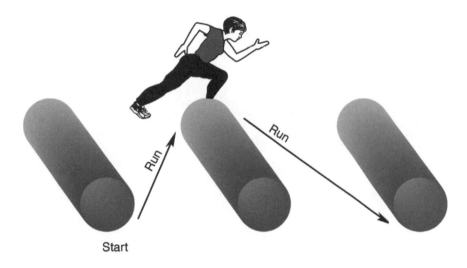

Change of Direction

Bag Drills

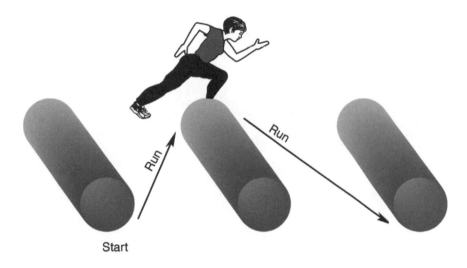

Run

Run

Start

PURPOSE

Development of change of direction and quick foot action

PROCEDURE

- Start in a two-point stance.
- Begin at one end of the bags on the right side and sprint forward toward the left side of the next bag.
- Planting the outside foot at the end of the bag, use a side-step to explosively propel forward toward the opposite end of the next bag.
- Complete the sprint through all the bags.

COMPLEX VARIATION

- Change distance between bags, as well as their orientation.
- Perform various biomotor skill combinations during the drill.

80

Bag Weave

Bag Drills

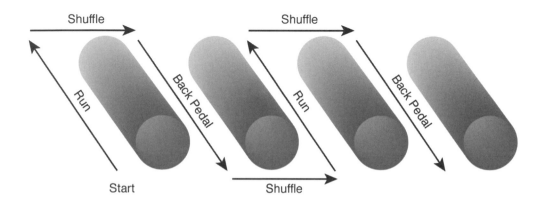

PURPOSE

Development of flexibility, high knee action, and quick foot action

PROCEDURE

- Start in a two-point stance.
- Starting on the outside of the first of 4 bags, sprint forward until you are in front of the bag.
- Shuffle the feet to the right until you reach a space between the bags, but do not cross the feet when moving sideways.
- Backpedal quickly until you are one step past the bag.
- Shuffle the feet again until you reach the outside of the last bag. Remember to always keep your shoulders square and to stay in a two-point stance while keeping your head up; use good running form while moving as fast as possible.

Combo Side Step/Forward Back

Bag Drills

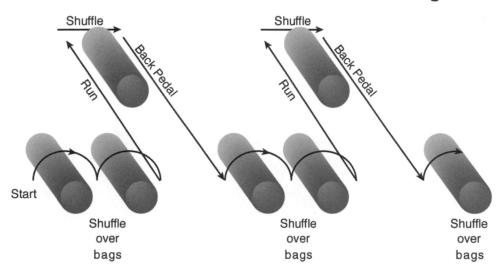

PURPOSE

Development of change of direction, flexibility, high knee action, and quick foot action

PROCEDURE

- Start in a two-point stance with hands and arms away from the body.
- Sprint laterally over the first two bags.
- Sprint 5 yards to the front of a third bag and shuffle.
- Backpedal 5 yards and laterally step over bags four and five.
- Sprint 5 yards to the front of the sixth bag and shuffle.
- Backpedal 5 yards and laterally step over bag seven.

COMPLEX VARIATION

- Combine skills to make drill more sport- or position-specific.

Agility

82

Lateral Weave

Bag Drills

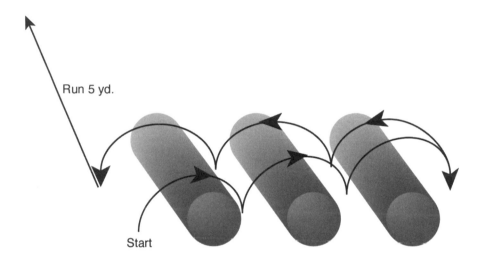

Run 5 yd.

Start

PURPOSE

Quick foot action and reaction development

PROCEDURE

- Start in a two-point stance with your hands and arms away from body.
- Laterally side-step over three or four bags quickly to the right or left.
- After crossing the last bag, immediately reverse directions.
- Once you cross the last bag, sprint forward 5 yards.

Agility

Bag Jumps With 180-Degree Turn

Bag Drills

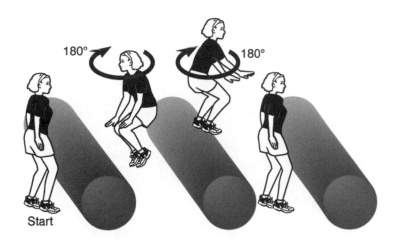

180°   180°

Start

Agility

PURPOSE

Foot quickness and kinesthetic awareness while providing explosive lower body development

PROCEDURE

- Start in a two-point stance.
- Laterally jump over the first bag, rotating 180 degrees while in the air.
- Land between two bags and immediately jump over the second bag, rotating 180 degrees in the opposite direction.
- Jump and rotate over 4 to 6 bags.

84

Wheel

Bag Drills

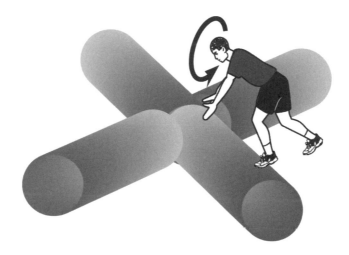

PURPOSE

Balance and quick foot action

PROCEDURE

- Arrange four bags in an X format.
- With both hands in the middle of the X formed by the bags, stand between two of the bags.
- Start by side-stepping over each bag while rotating around all 4 bags, keeping your hands in contact with the X formed by the bags until you are back at the original starting position.
- Quickly reverse directions and rotate back, side-stepping quickly over all 4 bags.

COMPLEX VARIATION

- Finish the drill by quickly sprinting 5 yards straight ahead out of the bags.

85

Crossover Step

Angle-Board Drills

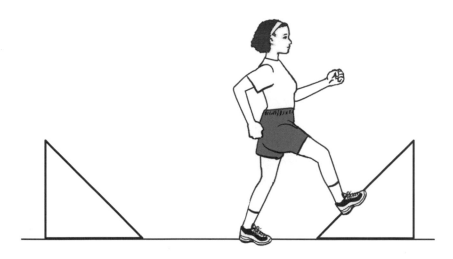

PURPOSE

Development of agility and rotation change of direction

PROCEDURE

- Start in a two-point stance on the run of the side strike.

- Cross the right foot over and strike the left angle.

- Shuffle with the left foot, bringing the right foot back to its original position.

- Cross the left foot over and strike the right angle.

- Shuffle with the right foot, bringing the left foot back to its original position.

- Repeat.

Agility

115

86

Cross-Behind Step

Angle-Board Drills

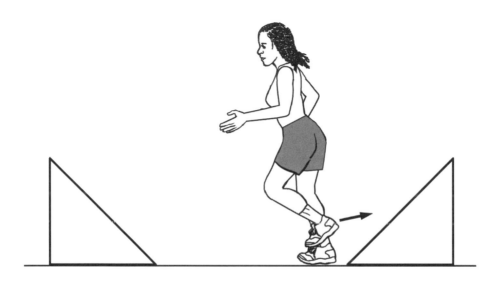

PURPOSE

Development of agility and rotation change of direction

PROCEDURE

- Start in a two-point stance on the run of the side strike.
- Cross the right foot behind the left and strike the left angle.
- Shuffle with the left foot, bringing the right foot back to its original position.
- Cross the left foot behind the right and strike the right angle.
- Shuffle with the right foot, bringing the left foot back to its original position.
- Repeat.

One Side Skier

Angle-Board Drills

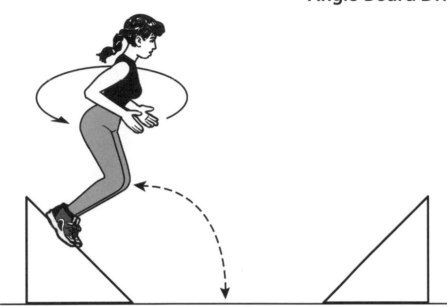

PURPOSE

Develop agility and rotational mechanics

PROCEDURE

- Start in a two-point stance on the run of the side strike, facing perpendicular to the side strike.

- Jump and rotate 90 degrees so as to land with both feet on the side angle.

- Jump back to land in the original position.

88

Side-to-Side Skiers

Angle-Board Drills

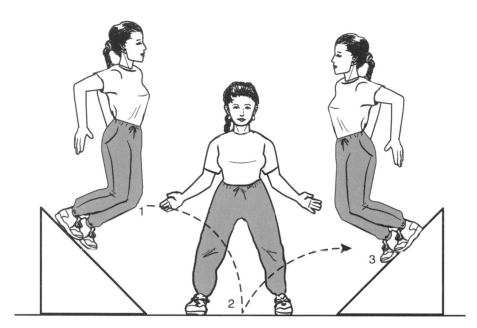

PURPOSE

Development of agility and rotation change of direction

PROCEDURE

- Start in a two-point stance on the run.

- The athlete stands perpendicular to the angles in the middle of the run.

- He or she jumps and rotates in midair so as to land with both feet on the right angle and facing the run. Immediately, he or she jumps back rotating in midair to land in the original position.

- The athlete jumps and rotates in midair so as to land with both feet on the left angle and facing the run. Immediately, he or she jumps back rotating in midair to land in the original position.

- Repeat.

Side-to-Side With Cone Reach

Slide Board Drills

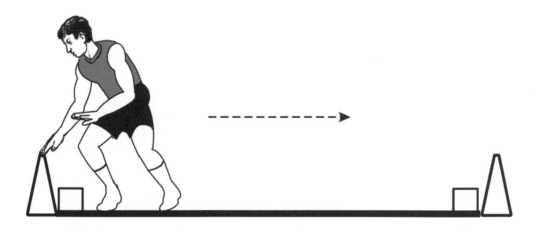

PURPOSE

Lateral agility, rotational transition, and balance

PROCEDURE

- Place a cone on each side of the slide board.
- Start in a two-point stance with a slight bend in the knees.
- Drop into a slight squat.
- Push off the slide board side support and glide to your right side.
- When you reach the right side, touch the cone with your outside hand.
- When you make contact with the cone, push off again and repeat.

COMPLEX VARIATION

- Use inside hand to touch cone.
- Perform sport-specific skill while sliding.

Agility

90

Front to Back

Slide Board Drills

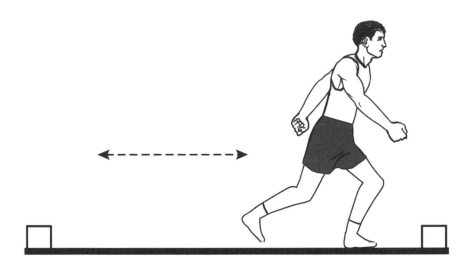

PURPOSE

Decelerative agility and balance

PROCEDURE

- Start in a two-point stance at one of the ends of the slide board with both feet on the side support.
- Stand with a slight bend in the knees.
- Drop into a slight squat and move the right leg forward as you push off the side support with the left.
- Stay in a lunge position with the right foot forward as you glide toward the other end.
- When your right foot touches, immediately push off again.
- Glide backwards in a lunge position and touch with the left foot.
- Repeat.
- Remember: keep opposite arm and leg movement through drill.

Side-to-Side With Front Rotation

Slide Board Drills

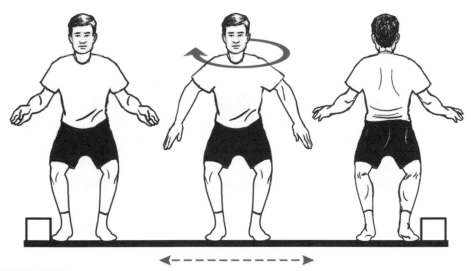

PURPOSE

Lateral agility, rotational transition, and balance

PROCEDURE

- Start in a two-point stance with a slight bend in the knees.
- Drop into a slight squat.
- Push off the slide board's side support and glide to the opposite side.
- While in transition, rotate counterclockwise so as to land on the opposite support with the push-off foot.
- When you make contact, push off again and repeat.
- Perform this drill to both the right and the left side.

Agility

Side-to-Side With Back Rotation

Slide Board Drills

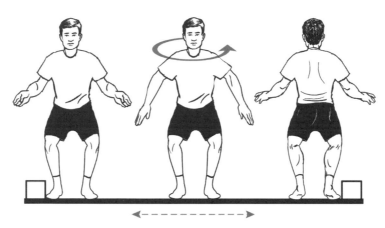

PURPOSE

Lateral agility, rotational transition, and balance

PROCEDURE

- Start in a two-point stance with a slight bend in the knees.
- Drop into a slight squat and swing the right leg behind in a speedskating fashion.
- Push off the slide board side support and glide to the opposite side.
- While in transition, rotate clockwise so as to land on the opposite support with the push-off foot.
- When you make contact, push off again and repeat.
- Perform drills to both the right and the left side.

Side-to-Side With Front and Back Combination

Slide Board Drills

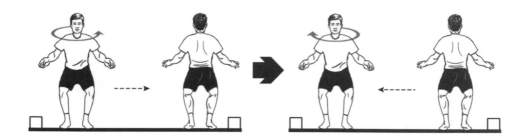

PURPOSE

Lateral agility, rotational transition, and balance

PROCEDURE

- Start in a two-point stance with a slight bend in the knees.

- Drop into a slight squat.

- Push off the slide board's side support and glide to the opposite side.

- While in transition, rotate clockwise so as to land on the opposite support with the push-off foot.

- When you make contact, push off the slide board's side support and glide to the other side.

- Push off the slide board's side support and glide to the opposite side.

- While in transition, rotate counterclockwise so as to land on the opposite support with the push-off foot.

- When you make contact push off again and repeat.

- Perform drills to both the right and the left side.

Agility

Stand Up From Four Points

Reactive Stand-Up Drills

Agility

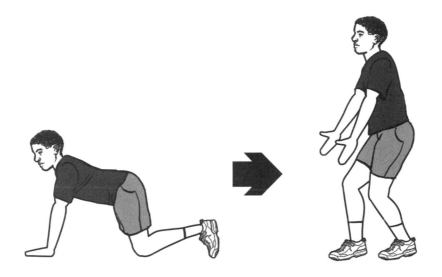

PURPOSE

Development of total body agility, kinesthetic awareness, and quickness

PROCEDURE

- Start on the ground on your hands and knees.
- Explode as you stand up as fast as possible.
- Use the following sequence: hands up, one foot up, then the other foot up.
- Repeat.

COMPLEX VARIATIONS

- React to a stimulus (e.g., whistle) and stand up.
- Follow stand up with sprint or sport-specific skill.

Stand Up From a Sitting Position

Reactive Stand-Up Drills

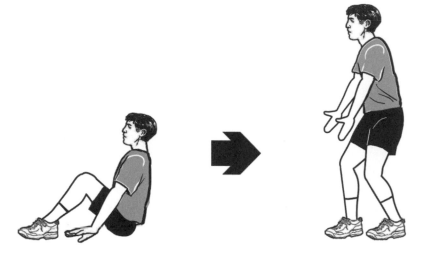

Agility

PURPOSE

Development of total body agility and kinesthetic awareness

PROCEDURE

- Start in a sitting position on the ground.
- Explode as you stand up as fast as possible.
- Practice rolling to either side to get up.
- Repeat.

COMPLEX VARIATION

- React to stimulus (e.g., whistle) and stand up.
- Follow with a sprint or sport-specific skill.

96

Stand Up From a Lying Position

Reactive Stand-Up Drills

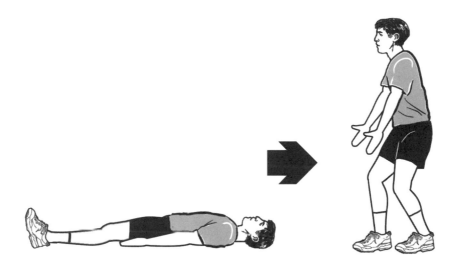

Agility

PURPOSE
  Development of total body agility and kinesthetic awareness

PROCEDURE
  • Start lying down in any position.
  • Stand up as fast as possible.
  • When facing up, practice rolling to either side to get up.
  • Repeat.

COMPLEX VARIATION
  • Start lying down in any position.
  • On command, stand up as fast as possible.
  • When facing up, practice rolling to either side to get up.
  • Follow with a sprint or sport-specific activity.

Sprawl and Stand Up

Reactive Stand-Up Drills

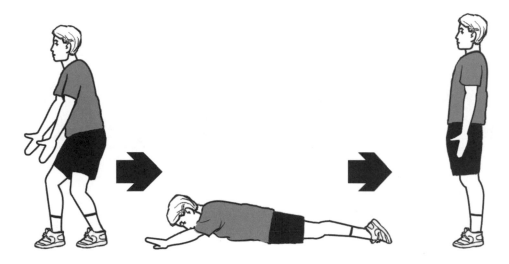

Agility

PURPOSE

Development of total body agility and kinesthetic awareness

PROCEDURE

- Start in a two-point stance.
- Perform a squat thrust, then a roll, and then get up as fast as possible.

COMPLEX VARIATION

- Roll after sprawling then stand up.
- Add a sprint or sport-specific activity after standing up.
- Add a biomotor skill (e.g., backpedal) after standing up.

98

Forward Roll Over Shoulder

Tumbling Drills

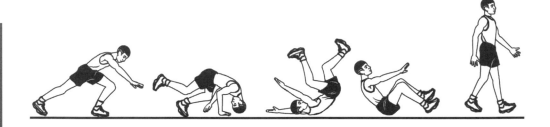

PURPOSE

Development of total body agility and kinesthetic awareness

PROCEDURE

- Start in a two-point stance with the left foot forward.
- Bend over and start to fall forward.
- As you are about to make contact with the ground, roll over the left shoulder.
- Roll and come back up to your feet.
- Perform forward rolls over both shoulders and with either foot forward.

COMPLEX VARIATION

- Add sprint in any direction after or before tumbling drill.
- React to any stimuli after tumbling (e.g., visual cue to run to a cone).
- Add a sport-specific skill after tumbling.

Agility

Backward Roll Over Shoulder

Tumbling Drills

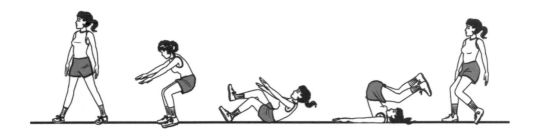

PURPOSE

Development of total body agility and kinesthetic awareness

PROCEDURE

- Start in a two-point stance.

- Bend the legs and start to sit on the ground behind you.

- As you are about to make contact with the ground, roll back over the left shoulder.

- Continue to roll and come back up to your feet.

- Perform backward rolls over both shoulders.

COMPLEX VARIATION

- Add sprint in any direction after or before tumbling drill.

- React to any stimuli after tumbling (e.g., visual cue to run to a cone).

- Add a sport-specific skill after tumbling.

Agility

100

Backward Roll to Hand Push-Off

Tumbling Drills

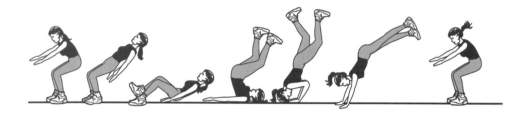

PURPOSE

Development of total body agility and kinesthetic awareness

PROCEDURE

- Start in a two-point stance.
- Bend the legs and start to sit on the ground behind you.
- As you are about to make contact with the ground, roll back.
- Continue to roll, and as your feet come over your head, press off using your hands and land on your feet.

COMPLEX VARIATION

- Add sprint in any direction after or before tumbling drill.
- React to any stimuli after tumbling (e.g., visual cue to run to a cone).
- Add a sport-specific skill after tumbling.

Agility

Forward Roll/Backward Roll Combination

Tumbling Drills

Agility

PURPOSE

Development of total body agility and kinesthetic awareness

PROCEDURE

- Start in a two-point stance.

- Perform a forward roll to your feet.

- Immediately go into a backward roll with a hands push-off.

- You may start and end this drill on your knees to reduce amplitude and difficulty.

COMPLEX VARIATION

- Add sprint in any direction after or before tumbling drill.

- React to any stimuli after tumbling (e.g., visual cue to run to a cone).

- Add a sport-specific skill after tumbling.

102

Cartwheel

Tumbling Drills

Agility

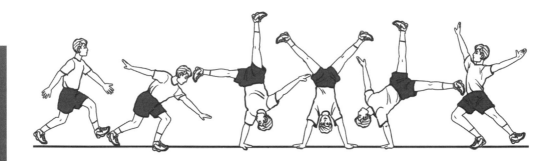

PURPOSE

Development of total body agility and kinesthetic awareness

PROCEDURE

- Start in a two-point stance.
- Laterally flex to the left and put your left hand on the ground.
- Continue to turn, putting your right hand on the other side of the left hand.
- As your feet go over you, the right foot lands and then the left foot lands on the other side.
- Perform drill to both sides.

COMPLEX VARIATION

- Add sprint in any direction after or before tumbling drill.
- React to any stimuli after tumbling (e.g., visual cue to run to a cone).
- Add a sport-specific skill after tumbling.

Round-Off

Tumbling Drills

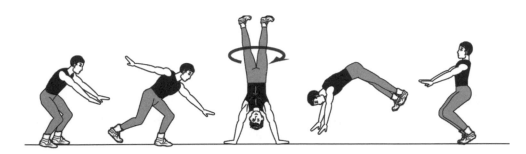

Agility

PURPOSE

Development of total body agility and kinesthetic awareness

PROCEDURE

- Start in a two-point stance.
- Laterally flex to the left and put your left hand on the ground.
- Continue to turn, putting your right hand on the other side of your left hand while bringing your feet over you.
- As your feet go over you, rotate your body and land with both feet facing the starting position.
- Perform drill to both sides.

COMPLEX VARIATION

- Add sprint in any direction after or before tumbling drill.
- React to any stimuli after tumbling (e.g., visual cue to run to a cone).
- Add a sport-specific skill after tumbling.

104

Running Start and Tumbling Over Barrier

Tumbling Drills

PURPOSE

Development of total body agility and kinesthetic awareness

PROCEDURE

- Perform all of the above drills with a running start and over a barrier.
- This will increase the amplitude and difficulty of the drill.

COMPLEX VARIATION

- Add sprint in any direction after or before tumbling drill.
- React to any stimuli after tumbling (e.g., visual cue to run to a cone).
- Add a sport-specific skill after tumbling.

Agility

Tumbling Sequencing

Tumbling Drills

PURPOSE
Development of total body agility and kinesthetic awareness

PROCEDURE
- String two or more of the tumbling drills together.
- This will increase the kinesthetic demands of the drill by requiring additional coordination and kinesthetics.

COMPLEX VARIATION
- Add sprint in any direction after or before tumbling drill.
- React to any stimuli after tumbling (e.g., visual cue to run to a cone).
- Add a sport-specific skill after tumbling.

Agility

Z-Ball 21 Drill

Crazy Z-Ball Drills

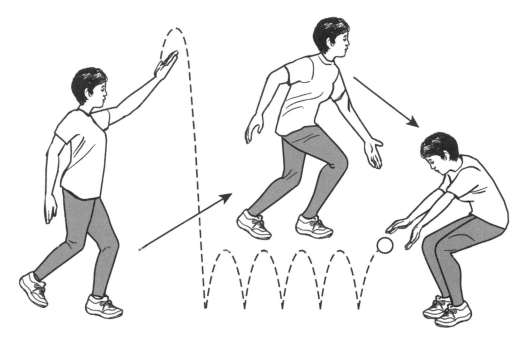

Agility

PURPOSE

Change of direction and reaction development

PROCEDURE

- Throw the Crazy Z-ball up in the air.

- Let it bounce as many time as you can while counting bounces.

- Catch it before it goes into a roll and award yourself the number of bounces as points.

- The first person to get to exactly "21" wins.

Drop and Get Up

Crazy Z-Ball Drills

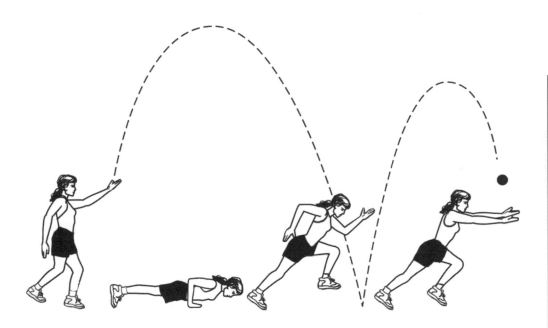

Agility

PURPOSE

Change of direction and reaction development

PROCEDURE

- Throw the Crazy Z-ball up in the air.
- Get onto the ground, perform a push-up, and get to the ball before the second bounce.
- This can be done after the first bounce.
- This can also start with a partner releasing the ball and the athlete on the ground.

108

Under and Go

Crazy Z-Ball Drills

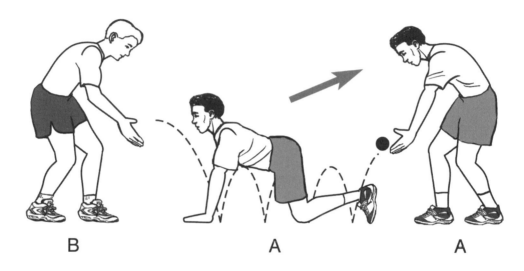

B   A   A

PURPOSE

Change of direction and reaction development

PROCEDURE

- Athlete "A" is on all fours.
- Athlete "B" passes the ball under athlete "A."
- Athlete "A" must get up and get the ball before it departs a marked area.
- This can also be done through the legs while standing in order to possess with feet or hands.

Hexagon Drill

Hex and Dot Drills

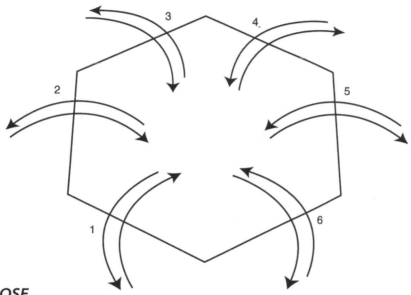

PURPOSE

Improve agility

PROCEDURE

- Each side of hexagon is about two feet long, though this can vary.

- Using a hexagon pattern, have the athlete begin in the middle, facing a determined direction.

- Always facing that direction, the athlete jumps with two feet outside each side of the hexagon sides.

- This should be done in a clockwise and counterclockwise direction while being timed.

COMPLEX VARIATION

- Use single leg hops.

- Vary the size of the hexagon.

5-Dot Drill

Hex and Dot Drills

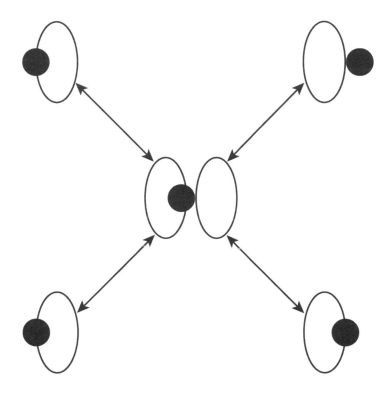

Agility

PURPOSE

Improving agility

PROCEDURE

- Using a 2-1-2 pattern of dots, create drills where predetermined patterns are performed for time.

- Patterns may include touching down with one foot only, two feet, or a combination.

Flip and Catch

Medicine Ball Drills

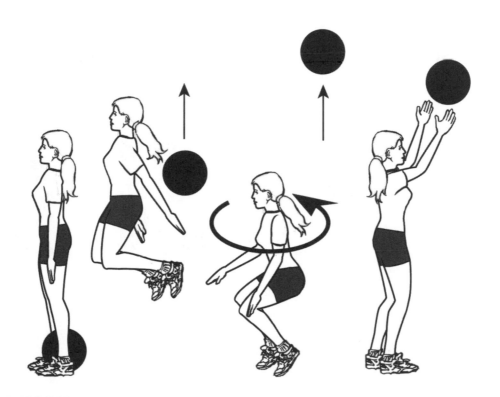

Agility

PURPOSE

Improve agility

PROCEDURE

- Start in a standing position, placing a medicine ball tightly between both feet.

- Proceed to jump into the air, kicking the ball into the air behind you.

- After landing, quickly turn and catch the ball before it hits the ground.

112

Toss, Get Up, and Catch

Medicine Ball Drills

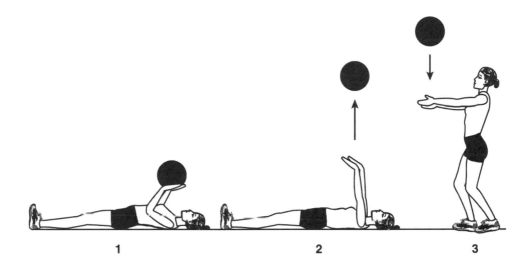

1   2   3

Agility

PURPOSE

Improve level change capability
Enhance transition from power to agility

PROCEDURE

- Lie down facing up.

- Hold a medicine ball in your hands.

- Perform a chest pass up in the air.

- Scramble up and catch the ball before it hits the ground.

REFERENCES

1. Arthur, M., and Bailey, B. Agility drills. Chapter 7 in *Complete Conditioning for Football* (pp. 191-237). Champaign, IL: Human Kinetics, 1998.

2. Barnes, M., and Attaway, J. Agility and conditioning of the San Francisco 49ers. *Strength and Conditioning* 18(4): 10-16, 1996.

3. Brittenham, G. Athleticism for basketball. Chapter 5 in *Complete Conditioning for Basketball* (pp. 69-87). Champaign, IL: Human Kinetics, 1996.

4. Costello, F., and Kreis, E.J. Introduction to agility. Chapter 1 in *Sports Agility* (pp. 2-3). Nashville, TN: Taylor Sports Publishing, 1993.

5. Fleck, S.J., and Kramer, W.J. *Designing Resistance Programs*, 2nd Edition. Champaign, IL: Human Kinetics, 1997.

6. Gambetta, V., and Myrland, S. *Speed/agility: Ladder footwork drills*. Gambetta Sports Training Systems, 1998.

7. Murphy, P., and Forney, J. Agility training. Chapter 7 in *Complete Conditioning for Baseball* (pp. 126-136). Champaign, IL: Human Kinetics, 1997.

8. Smythe, R. Acts of agility. *Training and Conditioning* V(4): 22-25, 27, 1995.

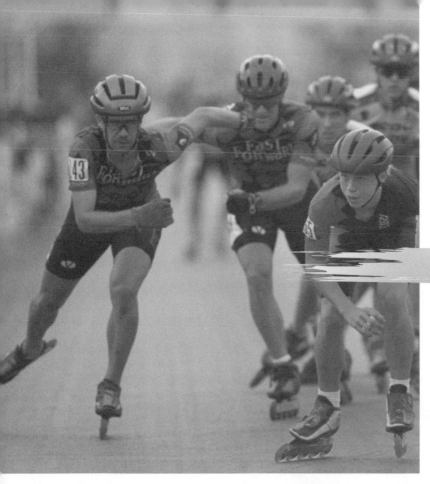

Quickness Training

Ian Pyka, MS, CSCS
Diane Vives, BS, CSCS

The successful performance of an athlete relies heavily on his or her ability to react quickly. Whether it be reacting to the auditory stimulus of a starter's pistol at the beginning of a race, out-jumping an opponent for a rebound on the basketball court, or being able to juke a defender on the football field, the quicker athlete usually maintains a competitive advantage.

"Quick," as defined by Webster, means:

- Reacting to a stimulus with *speed*
- Done or taking place with *rapidity*
- Marked by *speed*, readiness, promptness of physical movement
- Moving swiftly, occurring in a short time, responding to or understanding something *rapidly*

Speed, rapidity, and instancy are all words that are associated with quickness. One common theme to all of these descriptions is "rate" or the measure of something to a fixed unit. In this case, that fixed unit is time. When an athlete performs a task or movement in a relatively brief period of time, he or she can be described as being *quick*.

Quickness, in and of itself, seems simple enough to explain. An athlete is either quick or not, right? Wrong! Although it is true that genetic potential plays an important role in an athlete's physical abilities, many biomotor skills that depend on quickness may be improved.

When discussing quickness, we all have a tendency to discuss speed, acceleration, or agility in the same breath. "Did you see how *quickly* he accelerated?" we say, or, "Amazing how *quickly* she made those cuts!" and "Notice the *quick* leg turnover in that sprinter." All these characteristics are interconnected to some degree with quickness. But, are they components of quickness, or is quickness a mandatory requirement to enhance these characteristics needed for successful athletic performance?

"Reaction time," which is predicated on one's ability to react quickly to a stimulus, also plays a major role in many sports. How quickly a hockey player can react to the drop of a puck will determine what percentage of face-offs that player can win. Can we improve our reaction time?

In this chapter, we will attempt to answer these questions and discuss how sport-specific quickness can be improved. Finally, we will present the exercises and drills, from simple to complex, that we recommend to improve quickness for any sports-related movement.

QUICKNESS AND SKILL DEVELOPMENT

Athletes perform certain biomotor skills with an end result or purpose in mind. These "rehearsed" skills are recorded as patterns of motor movements in the brain. These recorded memories are referred to as neural *en-*

grams. In order to reproduce movement, the athlete calls on these engrams, which signal the motor system of the brain to reproduce the pattern.

If performed slowly, even highly complex motor skills can be accomplished the first time (i.e., learning). The movement must be slow enough at first to allow sensory feedback to occur and permit the proper adjustments necessary to guide a successful skill.

However, when faced with learning quick athletic movements, one must eventually perform the biomotor patterns associated with the movement as fast as possible. Successfully learning these motor skills is best achieved by successive and correct performance of the same activity.

New movements will always take a bit longer to correctly execute, while their patterns are recorded as a neural engram. Once the engram has been developed, it can then be recalled and performed with increasing effectiveness and proficiency. This certainly explains how an athlete who has performed a skilled movement countless times can do it so effortlessly and in a relaxed state. This relaxed and "second nature" quality is paramount to enhancing reaction and response time.

REACTION TIME

One of the definitions of *quick* was "reacting to a stimulus with speed." Interestingly, one definition of *reaction* is "bodily response to or an activity aroused by a stimulus." Webster also defines speed as "quickness or rapid motion." It should be clear once again that "quickness" is related to speed, time, and reaction. The time it takes an athlete to react to a stimulus may mean the difference between winning and losing.

Reaction time may involve auditory or visual senses, it may involve upper or lower extremities, or, in some cases, it may involve all of the above. An ice hockey goalie, for example, must be able to react to a hockey puck being shot at him at very high velocity. Initially, he spots the puck visually and reacts by blocking its path to the goal by using his legs, arms, or both.

Offensive football players react to the cadence of the quarterback's auditory signals, but the defensive players react to the exchange of the ball from center to quarterback. Reaction time to both simple and complex situations must be made all the time in sports. Reaction time is a determining factor in most sports and may be improved with training.[2]

SPEED AND ACCELERATION

A speed exercise is any exercise when quickness and high frequency are maximized. Speed and acceleration are both affected by quickness. One can increase running speed by increasing the stride frequency, which can be enhanced by "quicker" leg turnover. The ability of an athlete to accelerate also depends on increasing the quickness of limb movement, be it upper or lower body segments.

When the athlete learns the keys to initiating the movement (i.e., the starter gun or the snap of football), along with the sequential movement to follow (i.e., exploding from the starting blocks or engaging the opponent at the line of scrimmage), he or she can now concentrate more on movement output than sensory input. At this point, the athlete can work on moving from the slower learning of a sequence of movements to the faster "real time" sport-related skills themselves. Mastering the movement pattern first allows the athlete to concentrate on speed of movement or quickness.

SUMMARY

Improving quickness has major implications for the enhancement of speed, acceleration, and reaction time. The faster one can teach the brain the movement pattern required, the faster one can concentrate on improving the quickness with which that movement is performed, especially for new skills. Learning to be quicker is relatively simple. The key? Perform successive repetitions of technically correct movement patterns as fast as possible.

Now that you have been introduced to "quickness," let's find out how to become quicker. The following is a compilation of quickness exercises and drills that should help you gain that competitive edge.

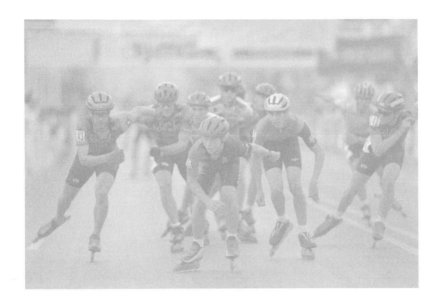

Drills for
Quickness Development

Although there is an obvious overlap between quickness, acceleration, and agility, we have tried to separate them into the "best" category to avoid duplication. Due to the overlap in the drills to develop each of these skills, some of the drills could have just as easily been categorized in another section of this book.

For this chapter, we have concentrated on the first-step reaction and on segmental acceleration. This section will also emphasize plyometrics involving reflex and reaction variables. The agility section will emphasize the transitional movements involved in quick level changes and fluid changes in body position. The speed section will emphasize locomotive acceleration and transition between running gears.

113

Backpedal

Assorted Biomotor Skills

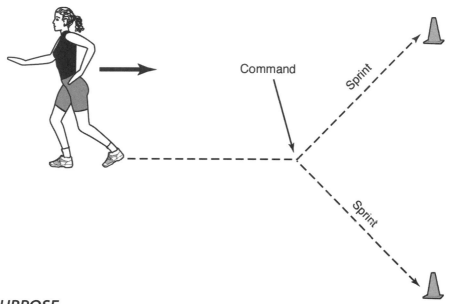

PURPOSE
Improve quickness and flexibility in the hip flexors

PROCEDURE
- In an athletic stance maintain your center of gravity over your base of support and run backwards.
- Increase stride length with good form.

COMPLEX VARIATION
- On command, use an "open step" and sprint to a designated cone.

Quickness

Multi-Directional Skipping

Assorted Biomotor Skills

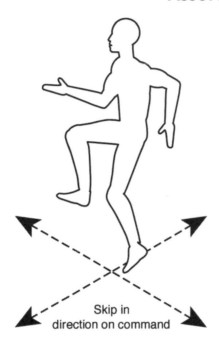

Skip in
direction on command

PURPOSE

Improve quickness and coordination in locomotive mechanics

PROCEDURE

- While skipping respond to commands or cues to change your direction, using forward, backward, and side skipping.

- Stay facing a target in front of you.

COMPLEX VARIATION

- Increase amplitude of skip and lower the number of reps.

- Concentrate on the first skip after the command to change direction.

- Add a sprint or skill on command.

Quickness

115

Side Shuffle

Assorted Biomotor Skills

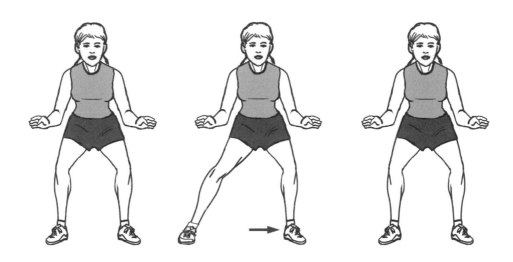

PURPOSE

Improve quickness in the lower body

PROCEDURE

- Begin in the athletic position.
- Shuffle inline in a determined direction without crossing the feet from point A to point B.
- This should be done by accelerating and then decelerating in order to stop as closely to point B as possible.
- Repeat this drill for time.

Quickness

Reaction Arm Sprints

Reaction Drills

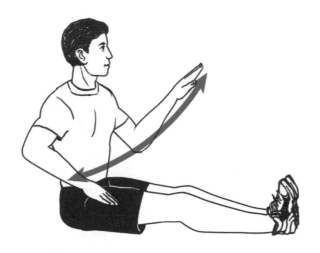

PURPOSE

Improve quickness in the upper body

PROCEDURE

- While seated on the ground, the athlete uses upper body running form and reacts on command for either a number of repetitions or a given time.

COMPLEX VARIATION

- Assume various positions (kneeling, standing, etc.).

- React to tactile, audio, or visual stimuli.

Quickness

117

Hot Hands

Reaction Drills

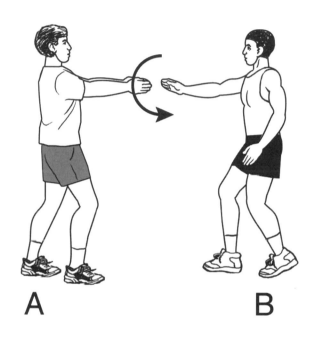

A   B

PURPOSE

Improve quickness in the upper body and reaction ability to visual stimuli

PROCEDURE

- Athlete "A" puts hands together (palm to palm) in front of himself or herself.

- Athlete "B" stands in front of athlete "A" with hands at his or her side.

- Athlete "B" tries to quickly touch (i.e., lightly slap) athlete "A's" hands while athlete "B" tries to react and avoid the contact.

Card Release

Reaction Drills

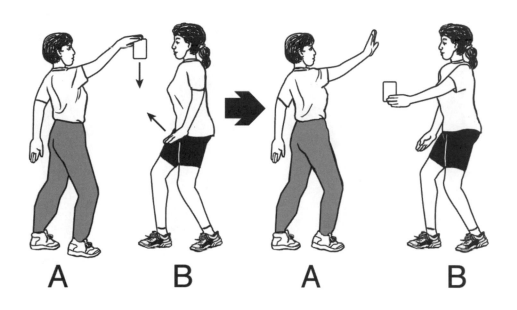

A   B   A   B

PURPOSE

Improve quickness in the upper body and reaction ability to visual stimuli

PROCEDURE

- Athlete "A" holds a playing card at shoulder height.
- Athlete "B" stands in front of athlete "A" in an athletic stance.
- Athlete "A" releases the card and athlete "B" reacts and attempts to catch it in midair.

Quickness

119

Card Snatching

Reaction Drills

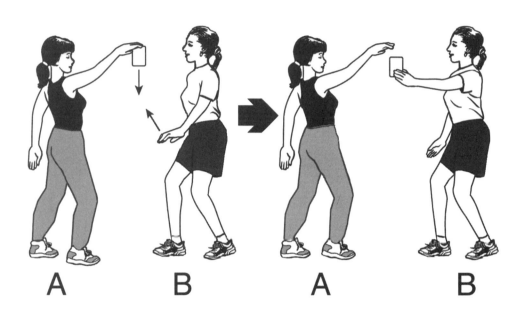

A   B   A   B

PURPOSE

Improve quickness in the upper body and reaction ability to visual stimuli

PROCEDURE

- Athlete "A" holds a playing card at shoulder height.
- Athlete "B" stands in front of athlete "A" in an athletic stance.
- Athlete "B" initiates the drill and attempts to snatch the card out of athlete "A"'s hand.
- Athlete "A" reacts and attempts to move the card so as to prevent athlete "B" from snatching it.

Quickness

The Bob (Slip)

Defensive Boxing Drills

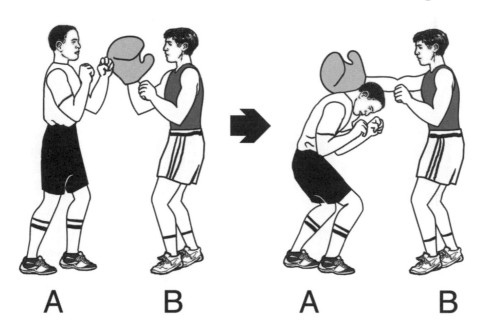

A   B   A   B

PURPOSE

Improve quickness of total body with upper body emphasis
Improve reaction time

PROCEDURE

- Athlete "A" get in an athletic stance particular to his or her sport or target technique.

- Athlete "B" stands in front of athlete "A."

- Using a foam bat, focus mitt, or an oversized boxing glove, athlete "B" initiates the drill by attempting to lightly contact the head area of athlete "A."

- The attack is made along the sagittal plane (i.e., straight on).

- Athlete "A" responds by slipping the attack (i.e., moving to either side of the attack).

Quickness

The Parry (Slap Block)

Defensive Boxing Drills

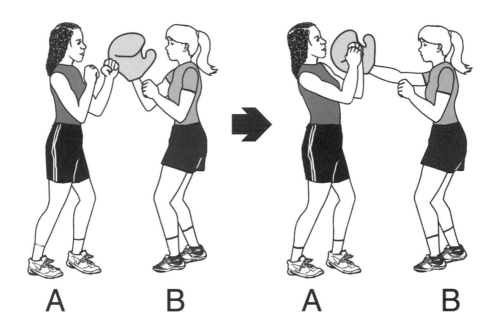

A   B   A   B

Quickness

PURPOSE

Improve quickness of total body with upper body emphasis
Improve reaction time

PROCEDURE

• Athlete "A" get in an athletic stance particular to his or her sport or target technique.

• Athlete "B" stands in front of athlete "A."

• Using a foam bat, focus mitt, or an oversized boxing glove, athlete "B" initiates the drill by attempting to lightly contact the head area of athlete "A."

• Athlete "A" responds by using his or her hands and slapping off the attack just before contact.

• The attack is made along the sagittal plane (i.e., straight on).

The Weave

Defensive Boxing Drills

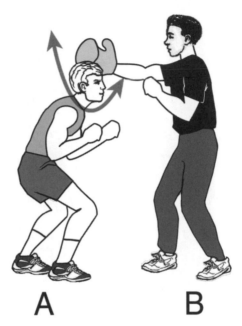

A   B

PURPOSE

Improve quickness in the upper body

PROCEDURE

- Athlete "A" get in an athletic stance particular to his or her sport or target technique.

- Athlete "B" stands in front of athlete "A."

- Using a foam bat, focus mitt, or an oversized boxing glove, athlete "B" initiates the drill by attempting to lightly contact the head area of athlete "A."

- The attack can be made along the sagittal or transverse plane (i.e., jab or roundhouse).

- Athlete "A" responds by weaving under the attack (i.e., ducking and weaving under the attack).

Quickness

123

Boxing Focus Mitt Simple Drills

Offensive Boxing Drills

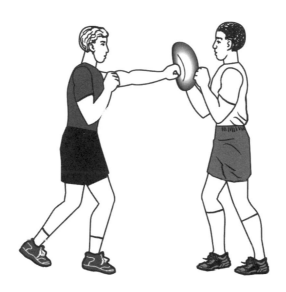

PURPOSE

    Improve reaction to visual stimulus
    Enhance hand and eye coordination

PROCEDURE

- Use the boxing focus mitts as a target.

- Present a mitt as a stimulus for the athlete to react to by using his or her hands to deliver a predetermined punch or slap to the focus mitt.

- This may be done to mimic sport-specific movements, such as the forehand in tennis or a hand technique used by football linemen.

Quickness

Boxing Focus Mitt Complex Drills

Offensive Boxing Drills

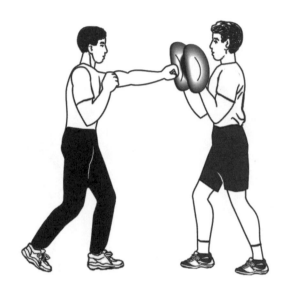

PURPOSE

Improve quickness in the upper body

PROCEDURE

- Teach the athlete two or more punches or responses.
- Present the focus mitt targets in a way that elicits a decision from the athlete.
- The athlete must deliver the correct response or combination of responses with quickness.

Quickness

125

Tap Drills (Simple Reaction Touches to a Target on Command)

Medicine Ball Reaction Drills

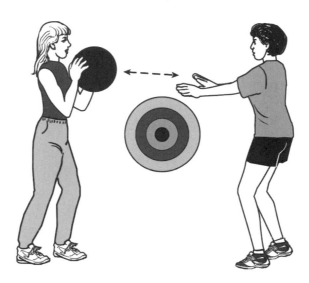

PURPOSE

Improve quickness in the upper body
Enhance elastic response of a pushing action

PROCEDURE

- Using a partner or trainer, the athlete reacts to the toss of a medicine ball and taps the ball to a target.
- The target location is decided prior to the toss.

COMPLEX VARIATION

- Provide various targets.
- Decide target location during the partner's toss.

One-Handed Tap Drills With Partner

Medicine Ball Reaction Drills

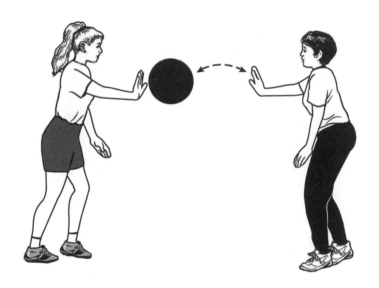

PURPOSE

Improve quickness and elastic upper body strength

PROCEDURE

- With arms extended, two athletes react to each other by tapping a medicine ball back and forth.

- Each touch uses a single hand, and the ball placement should progress to challenge your partner.

Quickness

127

Medicine Ball Bull in a Ring

Medicine Ball Reaction Drills

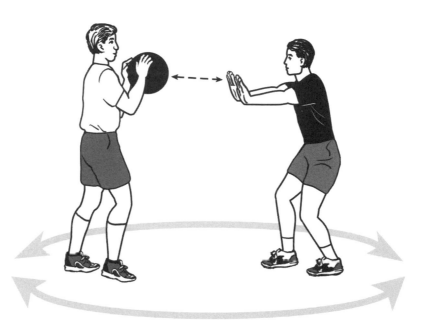

PURPOSE

Improve quickness and elastic strength

PROCEDURE

- Partners face each other and chest pass a medicine ball while staying in circle.

Quickness

Medicine Ball Lateral Shuffle/Pass

Medicine Ball Reaction Drills

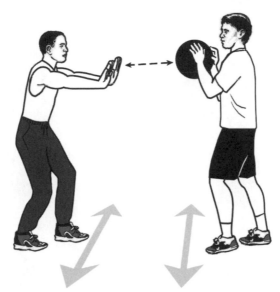

PURPOSE

Improve quickness and elastic strength

PROCEDURE

- This drill is performed with a partner and a medicine ball.
- The two athletes face each other.
- The distance depends on the weight of the medicine ball.
- The lighter the ball, the farther away the distance may become.
- The drill begins with both athletes shuffling laterally while performing a chest pass back and forth along the route.
- Upon reaching the target distance, the two return in the opposite direction while continuing to pass the ball.

COMPLEX VARIATION

- One athlete leads and is free to change direction at will.
- The other athlete reacts and follows.

Quickness

Mirror Lateral Shuffle/Pass

Medicine Ball Reaction Drills

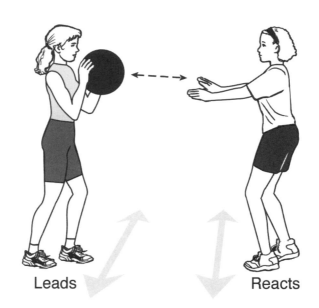

Leads   Reacts

PURPOSE

Improve quickness in the upper body

PROCEDURE

- Same as the Medicine Ball Lateral Shuffle/Pass, except that one athlete leads the drill by changing direction (left or right) in an attempt to lose the opponent.

- The drill can be limited by time.

- The shorter the time of the drill, the greater the intensity.

Quickness

Medicine Ball Squat, Push Toss, Bounce, and Catch

Medicine Ball Reaction Drills

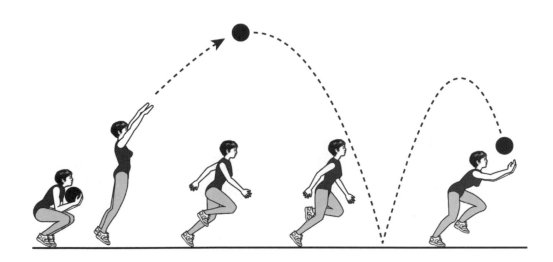

PURPOSE

Improve reactive and elastic strength and total body power

PROCEDURE

- This drill is performed with a rubber medicine ball that can bounce.

- The athlete begins by holding the ball chest high, squatting down then throwing the ball for height and distance.

- The athlete then has to be quick enough to chase after the ball and catch it before it bounces a second time.

- Obviously, a ball that is too light will travel too far, making it very difficult for the athlete to retrieve it in time.

Quickness

131

Medicine Ball Reverse Scoop Toss, Bounce, and Catch

Medicine Ball Reaction Drills

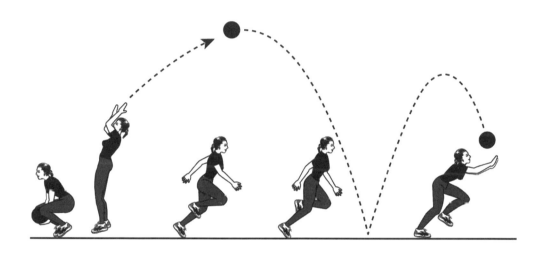

PURPOSE

Improve total body power and reactive strength

PROCEDURE

- The medicine ball is swung between the legs as the athlete squats down and then thrown overhead for height and distance.

- The athlete then turns and sprints toward the ball to attempt to catch it before the second bounce.

Quickness

Ball Drops With a Partner

Sports Ball Reaction Drills

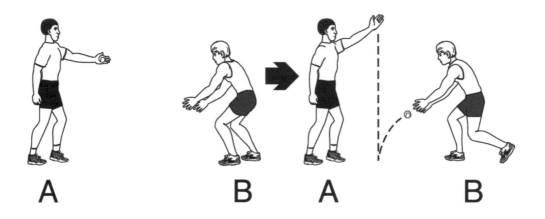

A   B   A   B

PURPOSE

Improve visual stimulus response and first-step quickness

PROCEDURE

- Using a ball, which can be specific to the target sport, have a partner stationed about 5 yards away and drop the ball from shoulder height.

- The retriever must catch the ball before the second bounce.

COMPLEX VARIATION

- The height of the drop, or distance between partners, can be changed to accommodate skill level.

- You may choose to use a ball in each hand in order to increase the difficulty of responding.

Quickness

133

Quick Hands Toss

Sports Ball Reaction Drills

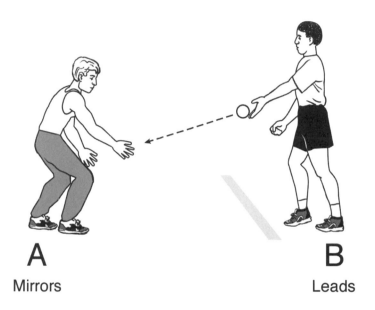

A	B
Mirrors	Leads

PURPOSE

Improve hand and eye coordination and quick change of direction

PROCEDURE

- Player "A" stands on a line in athletic ready position.
- Player "B" then tosses a tennis ball with either hand as player "A" reacts, catching the ball.

COMPLEX VARIATION

- Call out hand to be used to catch the ball.
- Require "mirror" and "opposite" hand catching patterns.

Dodge Ball

Sports Ball Reaction Drills

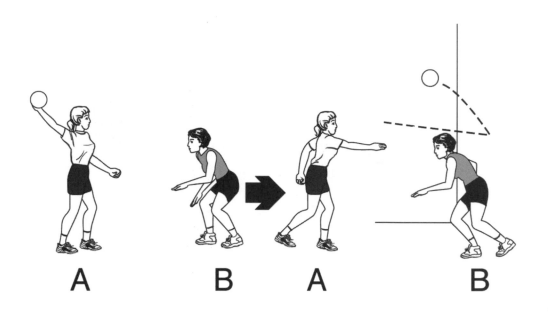

A   B   A   B

PURPOSE

Improve visual stimuli response and total-body quickness

PROCEDURE

- This game can be played against the wall with 2 to 4 players or in a circle with 5 or more players.

- Using a ball, which can be specific to the target sport (e.g., tennis ball, Nerf ball, volleyball, basketball), place one player up against a wall or inside the circle.

- The player against the wall or inside the circle attempts to evade the ball as it is thrown at him or her.

Quickness

135

Bounce and Catch

Sports Ball Reaction Drills

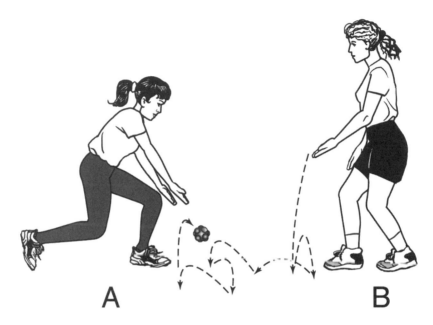

A   B

PURPOSE

Improve hand and eye coordination and first-step quickness

PROCEDURE

- Player "A" must stand in ready position as player "B" bounces the Crazy-ball on the ground.
- Player "A" catches the ball after it bounces one or two times.

COMPLEX VARIATION

- Player "A" must stand in ready position as player "B" bounces the Crazy Z-ball on the ground and calls out "1" or "2."
- Player "B" catches on the bounce number that has been called.
- Player "A" can also signal what hand to use to catch the crazy ball (e.g., "one-left," meaning catch on the first bounce with the left hand).

Quickness

136

Goalie Drill (Line Creates Boundary)

Sports Ball Reaction Drills

A   B

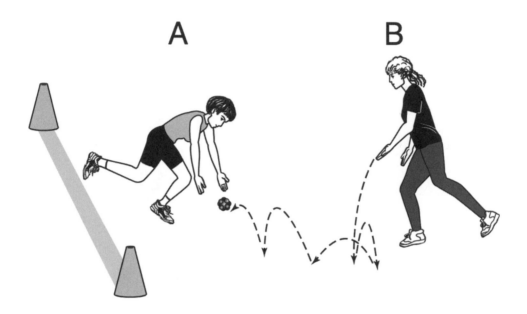

PURPOSE

Improve quickness in the upper body

PROCEDURE

- A line and cones define a goal.
- Player "A" is the goalie, and player "B" is the shooter.
- Player "B" rolls the ball towards the goal.
- Player "A" tries to stop the ball from crossing the line.
- The players can use hands, feet, or any combination to stop the ball from crossing the goal line.

Quickness

137

Stability Ball Cyclic Impact Lockouts

Stability Ball Reaction Drills

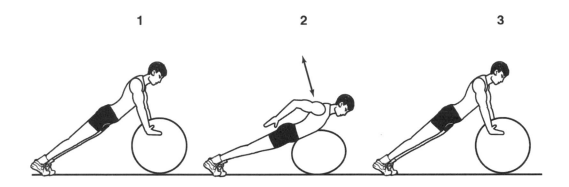

1   2   3

PURPOSE

Strengthen core and improve the body's ability to absorb impact

PROCEDURE

- Assume a "hand-on-ball" push-up position.
- Keep the core (abs, lower back, and hips) tight.
- Release the ball, allowing yourself to fall on the ball.
- Make impact on upper abdominals.
- As you bounce off the ball, secure the ball with the hands and lock-out the arms.

COMPLEX VARIATION

- Reach out and touch a target while bouncing.
- Clap your hands behind your body while bouncing.

Stability Ball Hops

Stability Ball Reaction Drills

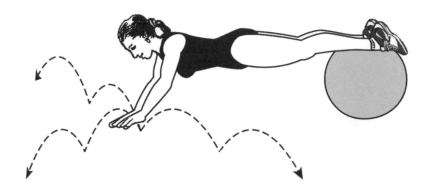

PURPOSE

Improve quickness in the upper-body pushing musculature

PROCEDURE

- Placing your feet on the stability ball and hands on the floor (push-up position), begin to hop backward and forward and from side to side, maintaining your balance on the ball with your feet.

- Do not allow the abdominals and hips to sag. Maintain a firm body position.

Quickness

139

Wheelbarrow Drill

Upper-Body Plyometric Drills

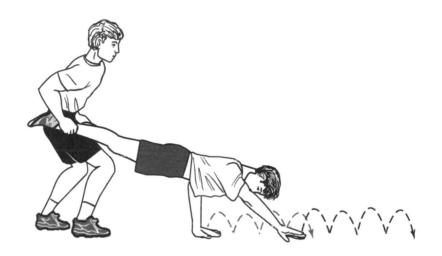

PURPOSE

Improve power in the upper body and core

PROCEDURE

- A partner holds an athlete's feet while his or her hands perform a predetermined pattern or task.
- This should be done as quickly as possible while maintaining a straight body.
- It can be timed to judge improvements, or you can encourage the use of visual cues such as ladders, mini-hurdles, dot patterns, and so on.

COMPLEX VARIATION

- Perform jumps instead of hand runs.
- Perform lateral shuffles or circular walks with hands.

Quickness

Plyo Push-Ups

Upper-Body Plyometric Drills

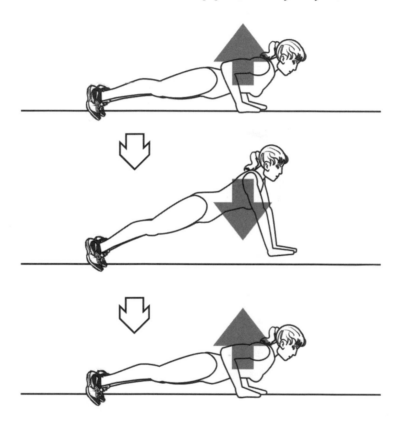

PURPOSE

Improve quickness in the upper-body pushing musculature

PROCEDURE

- Beginning in the up position, perform an explosive push-up. The hands should leave the ground, achieving as much space between the hands and the ground as possible. Finish with the arms extended.

- When landing, keep your arms stiff, but not locked. Spend as little time on the ground as possible, and explode back up.

Quickness

141

Medicine Ball Wall Chest Passes

Upper-Body Plyometric Drills

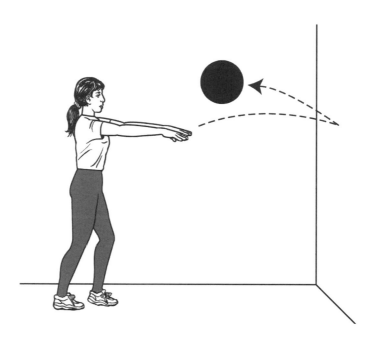

PURPOSE

Improve total body transmission of power

PROCEDURE

- Using the wall, the thrower performs chest passes to the wall and receives the ball with arms extended before performing the next pass.

- This can be done for any number of repetitions, for time, or for distance.

COMPLEX VARIATION

- Perform with one arm.

- Perform while moving laterally up and down the wall.

Quickness

Medicine Ball Release Push-Ups With Partner

Upper-Body Plyometric Drills

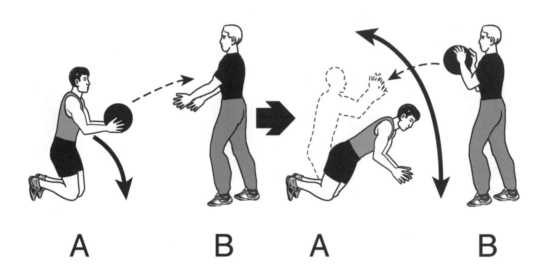

A   B   A   B

PURPOSE

Improve quickness in the upper-body pushing musculature

PROCEDURE

- Starting in a kneeling position, the athlete throws the medicine ball to a partner, then falls into a push-up.

- Pushing up back into the start position while the partner returns the medicine ball, the athlete repeats the exercise as quickly as possible.

Quickness

179

143

Medicine Ball Punches

Upper-Body Plyometric Drills

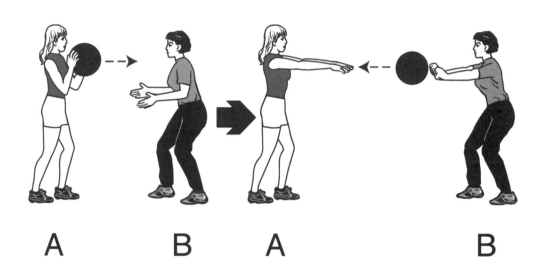

A   B   A   B

PURPOSE

Enhances total body power transmission

PROCEDURE

- A thrower tosses a ball at a receiver, and the receiver meets the ball with arms extended and punches the ball back to thrower.

- Change the rhythm to challenge the receiver.

- The receiver attempts to minimize contact time (i.e., amortization time) while producing maximum force.

COMPLEX VARIATION

- Both athletes can be moving laterally.

Quickness

Medicine Ball Wall Side Toss

Upper-Body Plyometric Drills

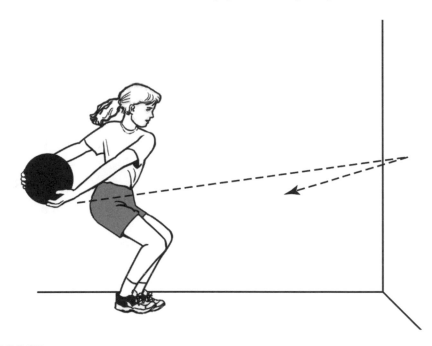

PURPOSE
Enhance explosive rotational mechanics and changes in direction

PROCEDURE
- Begin by facing the wall in an athletic position with a medicine ball held at your side.
- Throw the ball, striking the wall directly in front of you.

COMPLEX VARIATION
- Use different stances, such as perpendicular to the wall.
- Use parallel stance and toss the ball so that it rebounds to the other side of your body.

Quickness

145

Medicine Ball Overhead Throw

Upper-Body Plyometric Drills

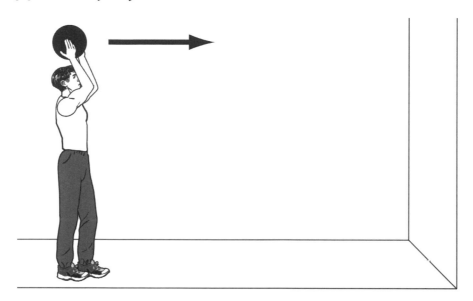

PURPOSE

Improve explosive power in throwing or overhead activities

PROCEDURE

- Using the wall, the athlete loads the ball over and behind the head, extending the entire body.
- Keep a parallel stance and feet flat during the loading or "cocking" phase.

COMPLEX VARIATION

- Step forward while throwing (alternate legs).
- Throw from a kneeling position.

Quickness

Medicine Ball Wall Scoop Toss

Upper-Body Plyometric Drills

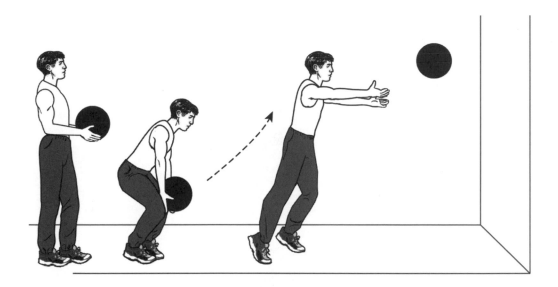

PURPOSE

Enhance total body extension, quickness, and power

PROCEDURE

- Face a wall in an upright athletic stance with a medicine ball.
- Quickly squat and extend your entire body.
- Toss the ball against the wall as fast as possible while maintaining a tight-backed, low-squat stance.
- Perform this drill for time or number of repetitions.

COMPLEX VARIATION

- Perform a reverse scoop toss backwards.
- Perform a long jump and then scoop toss.

Quickness

147

Foot-Tapping Frequency

Lower-Body Reaction Drills

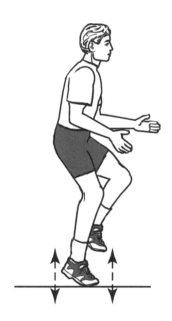

PURPOSE

Improve quickness in the lower body

PROCEDURE

- Stand with knees and hips slightly flexed, arms relaxed, and shoulders over toes, prepared to react to stimulus to start.

- On either a visual or auditory cue, begin to tap your feet alternately as fast as possible for a predetermined amount of time.

COMPLEX VARIATION

- Mirror another athlete or react to any form of stimuli.

- Perform laterally, forward, or diagonally.

- Add a sprint in any direction on cue.

Quickness

Directional Foot Movement

Lower-Body Reaction Drills

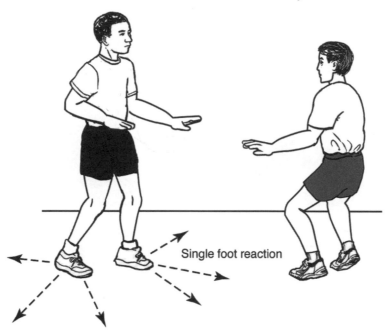

Single foot reaction

PURPOSE

Improve reactive quickness and first-step reaction

PROCEDURE

- Have the athlete move his or her foot in the direction of a stimulus (hand signal, ball toss, etc.).

- Work only on first-step reaction.

COMPLEX VARIATION

- Add a second step and eventually a sprint to follow the reaction.

- Add a skill after the reaction, or sprint.

Quickness

Directional Mirror Drill

Lower-Body Reaction Drills

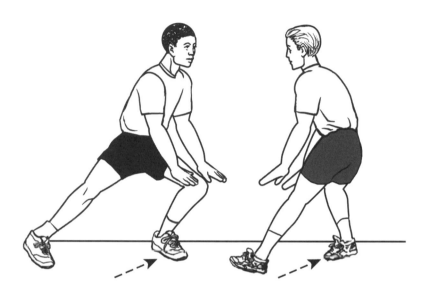

PURPOSE

Improve quickness in the lower body

PROCEDURE

- This drill is performed between partners.
- Perform all directional foot movement and variations.
- One partner initiates the leg movements, at which time the other partner reacts by trying to mirror the same movement.

Quickness

Sprint and Backpedal on Command

Reactive Running Drills

● Whistle

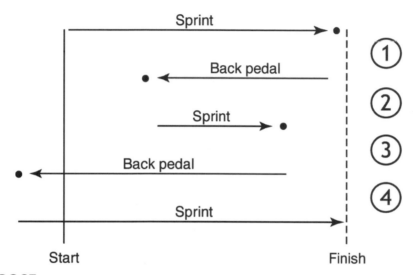

PURPOSE

Improve reaction and change of direction capabilities

PROCEDURE

- Start in two-point stance.
- On command, sprint.
- On next command, backpedal.
- Repeat.

COMPLEX VARIATION

- Start from different positions.
- Change biomotor skills throughout the drill, or for each command.
- Add a plyometric exercise at each command.
- Vary distances between commands.

Quickness

Sprint and Cut on Command

Reactive Running Drills

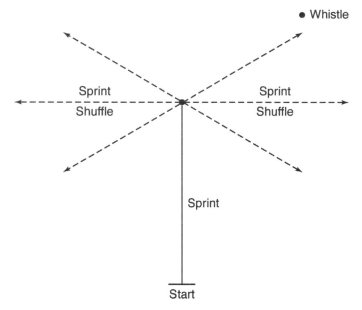

PURPOSE

Improve reaction time and change of direction capability

PROCEDURE

- Start in a two-point stance.
- Sprint on command, cut sharply, and sprint in the instructed direction.

COMPLEX VARIATION

- Start from different positions.
- Change biomotor skills throughout the drill, or for each command.
- Add a plyometric exercise at each command.
- Vary distances between commands.
- Change the cut angle.

Quickness

Backpedal and Cut on Command

Reactive Running Drills

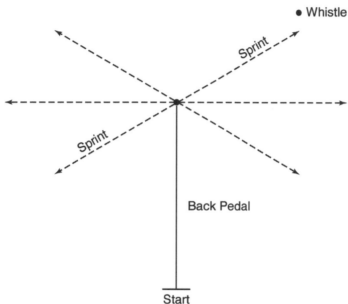

● Whistle

Sprint

Sprint

Back Pedal

Start

PURPOSE

Improve reaction time and change of direction ability

PROCEDURE

- Start in a two-point stance.
- Backpedal on command, cut sharply, and sprint to the designated direction.

COMPLEX VARIATION

- Start from different positions.
- Change biomotor skills throughout the drill, or for each command.
- Add a plyometric exercise at each command.
- Vary distances between commands.

Quickness

153

8-Point Star Drill

Reactive Running Drills

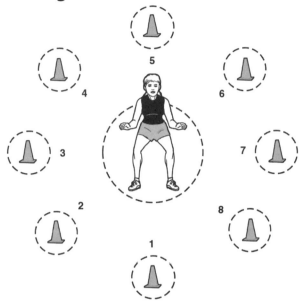

PURPOSE

Improve multi-directional first-step quickness and reaction time

PROCEDURE

- Stand in the middle of eight cones or circles (can use sidewalk chalk to draw them on a paved surface).

- Assume an athletic position and wait for a signal.

- React to the signal and run to each circle, putting one foot in each circle.

- Run back until both feet are on the inside circle.

- Perform drill in a clockwise and counterclockwise direction.

COMPLEX VARIATION

- Run around each cone or circle.

- Go to the cone or circle the coach calls out.

Quickness

154

Side Shuffle

Angle-Board Drills

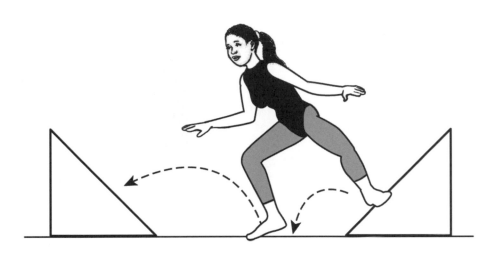

PURPOSE

Improve lateral first-step capability

PROCEDURE

- The athlete stands with the right foot on the right angle and the left foot on the flat run.

- He or she takes a short lateral step to the run with the left foot, then with the right foot.

- The left foot then hits the left angle.

- He or she then takes a short lateral step to the run with the right foot, then with the left foot.

- The right foot then hits the angle.

Note: All side-strike drills can be performed for time or foot contacts.

Quickness

155

Front Shuffle

Angle-Board Drills

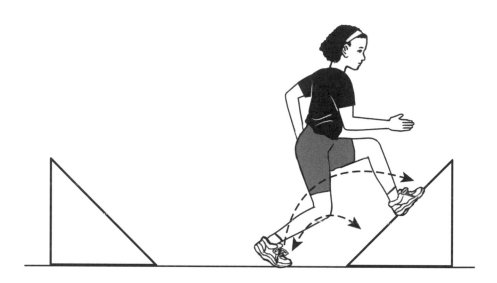

PURPOSE

Improve first-step capability

PROCEDURE

- The athlete stands with both feet on the run facing one of the angles.
- He or she takes a short forward step to the angle with the left foot, then shuffles with the right foot on the run.
- The left foot then steps on the run.
- Repeat with the right foot.

Quickness

Back Shuffle

Angle-Board Drills

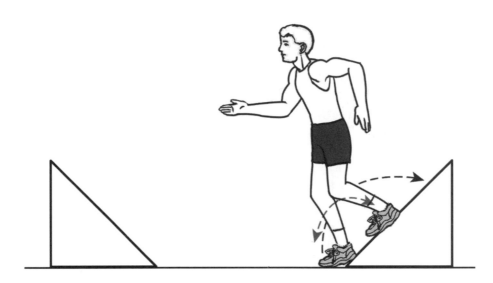

PURPOSE

Improve quickness in the lower body

PROCEDURE

- The athlete stands with both feet on the run facing away from one of the angles.
- He or she takes a short forward step back to the angle with the left foot, then shuffles with the right foot on the run.
- The left foot then steps on the run.
- Repeat with the right foot.

Quickness

157

Medicine Ball Between Leg Flips (Maravich)

Medicine Ball Explosive Drills

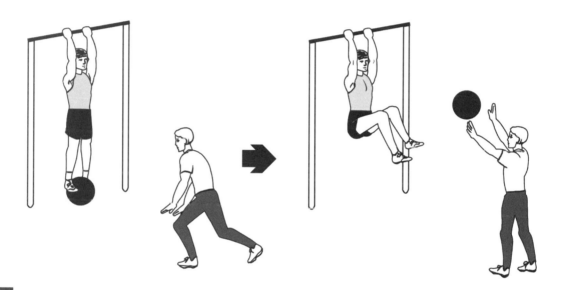

PURPOSE

Improve total body power

PROCEDURE

- The receiver hangs from a chin-up bar that allows the feet to touch the ground.
- A partner rolls the medicine ball to the receiver's feet.
- The receiver then picks up the ball between the feet and flips it back to the partner as quickly as possible.

Quickness

Pike Kick Up and Catch

Medicine Ball Explosive Drills

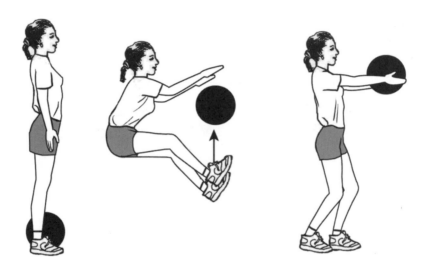

PURPOSE

Improve total body power

PROCEDURE

- The athlete holds the medicine ball between his or her feet, then explosively kicks the ball up and catches it in front.

Quickness

Quick Feet (in All Directions)

Half Agility Ladder Drills With Reaction Command

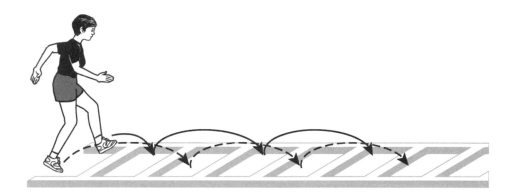

Quickness

PURPOSE

Enhance stride frequency at first step

PROCEDURE

- Run through an agility ladder using a "one foot down between each rung" pattern.

- Concentrate on foot speed not linear running speed.

- For variation, react to command and run to designated target.

Note: To avoid duplication, we have split the Agility Ladder Drills between this and the agility chapter. The following drills will emphasize short, "first-step" quickness. For this reason, the following drills will use half of a standard agility ladder. This will make the drill quicker and not allow neural fatigue to become a significant factor. Additionally, the reaction command will add the reaction/response component emphasized in this chapter.

The coach can designate predetermined cones (e.g., one cone on each side of the ladder, 5-10 yards from the ladder) for the athlete to run to upon receiving an audible or visual command. *Every drill can be performed laterally or backwards for increased difficulty.*

Skips

Half Agility Ladder Drills With Reaction Command

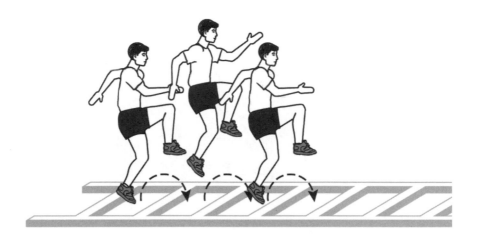

PURPOSE

Improve hip, leg, and ankle power

PROCEDURE

- Skip, using every rung.
- Skip in all directions (i.e., front, side, and back).
- Look straight ahead, not down.
- To add difficulty, a skill can be added to the drill.

Quickness

161

Side Step

Half Agility Ladder Drills With Reaction Command

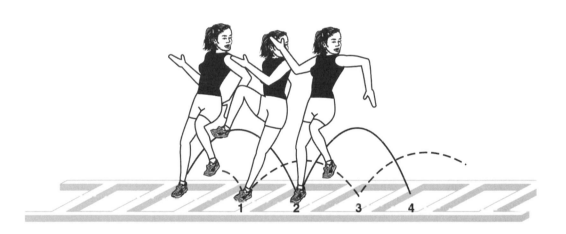

Quickness

PURPOSE

Development of balance, flexibility, footwork development, and peripheral vision

PROCEDURE

- Start in a two-point stance.
- Sprint laterally through the agility ladder using high knee and good arm action.
- Hit alternating feet in each square of the ladder.
- Look up, not at the ground.

Side Step/Double Step

Half Agility Ladder Drills With Reaction Command

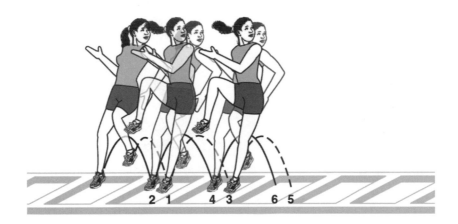

2 1   4 3   6 5

PURPOSE

Development of balance, flexibility, foot quickness, and peripheral vision

PROCEDURE

- Start in a two-point stance.
- Sprint laterally through the agility ladder using high knee and good arm action.
- Hit each foot in every square of the ladder.
- Look up, not at the ground.

Quickness

163

Bunny Jumps

Half Agility Ladder Drills With Reaction Command

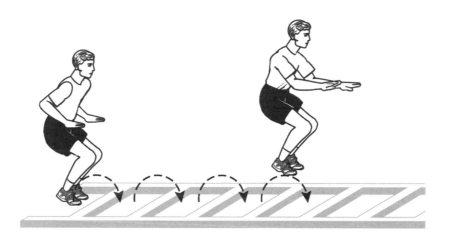

PURPOSE

Enhance elastic strength in the ankle complex

PROCEDURE

- Perform fast multiple jumps into every square of the ladder.
- Use quick ankling motion.
- Minimize ground contact.
- To add difficulty, a skill can be added to the drill.
- Look straight ahead, not at the ground.

Quickness

Hop-Scotch Drill

Half Agility Ladder Drills With Reaction Command

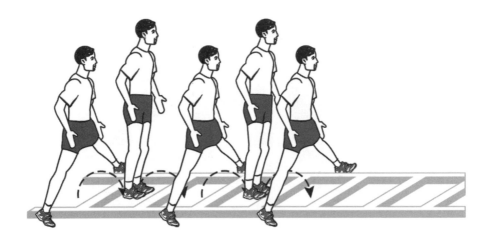

PURPOSE

Enhance elastic strength in the ankle complex

PROCEDURE

- Start with one foot on each side of the ladder.
- Jump with both feet into the first space, then jump to the next space. Spread feet apart so that each one lands on the outside of the ladder.
- Then jump with both feet into the next square on the ladder.
- Keep repeating.
- To add difficulty, a skill can be added to the drill.
- Look straight ahead, not at the ground.

COMPLEX VARIATION

- Land on one foot when landing inside the ladder squares.

Quickness

165

One-Leg Hop

Half Agility Ladder Drills With Reaction Command

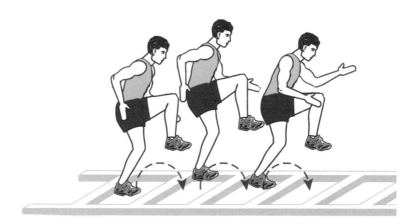

PURPOSE

Improve quickness in the lower body

PROCEDURE

- Hop in every square using only one leg.
- Emphasize minimizing ground contact.
- To add difficulty, a skill can be added to the drill.
- Look straight ahead, not at the ground.

Change of Skill

Half Agility Ladder Drills With Reaction Command

PURPOSE

Improve quickness in the lower body

PROCEDURE

- Have the athlete change skill (e.g., hop to skip) upon different cues (audio, visual, tactile).

- To add difficulty, a skill can be added to the drill.

Quickness

167

Half Ladder Skill to Sport-Specific Skill

Half Agility Ladder Drills With Reaction Command

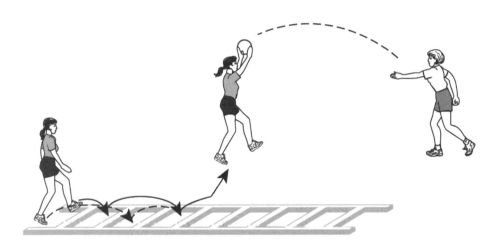

PURPOSE

Improve quickness in the lower body

PROCEDURE

- The athlete can perform any of the Agility Ladder Drills while looking at the coach, who is positioned at the opposite side of the ladder.

- The athlete reacts to the coach throwing a ball (e.g., a football, baseball, tennis ball, etc.) to either side of the ladder (e.g., right or left).

- The athlete reacts in mid-run to the side of the throw and catches or hits the ball.

Note: Combinations of biomotor skills are limitless—use your imagination.

168

Half Ladder Skill While Performing Sport-Specific Activity

Half Agility Ladder Drills With Reaction Command

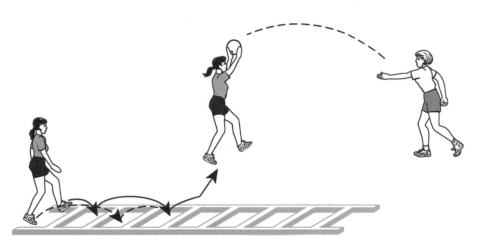

PURPOSE

Improve quickness in the lower body

PROCEDURE

- Perform any of the Agility Ladder Drills while performing any sport-specific activity.

- React to the coach throwing a ball (e.g., football, baseball, tennis ball, etc.) to you.

- React in mid-run and catch the ball or hit the ball back to the coach.

- Weighted medicine balls may be used to add difficulty to this drill.

Quickness

Rope-Skipping

Lower-Body Plyometric Drills

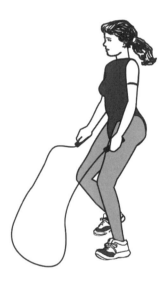

PURPOSE

Improve quickness and elastic strength in the lower body

PROCEDURE

- Skip rope while jumping to designated spots on the ground.
- This drill may be performed with both legs or a single leg.

VARIATIONS

- Variable Patterns—Skip rope while changing patterns to commands. This variation may be performed with double legs or a single leg.
- Weighted Rope Skipping—Perform the drill with a weighted rope.
- Side Skipping—Perform the drill to the left or right. The arm and knee sequence should remain the same throughout. This drill can be the most challenging of all the skips.

Quickness

In-Place Ankle Jumps

Lower-Body Plyometric Drills

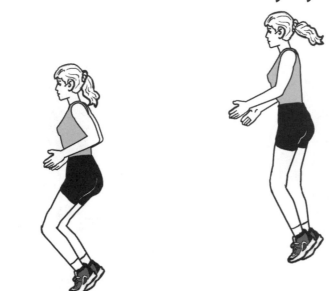

PURPOSE

Improve elastic strength and quickness in lower body

PROCEDURE

- Perform in-place jumps just using the ankle.
- Spend minimum amount of time on the ground.

COMPLEX VARIATION

- Jump over a line on the ground, back and forth or sideways.

Note: All plyometric exercises can be initiated via a stimulus (whistle, etc.), and can be preceded or followed by any skill (catching a ball, sprinting, tumbling, etc.).

Quickness

171

Hip-Twist Ankle Jumps

Lower-Body Plyometric Drills

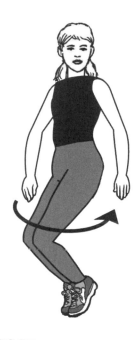 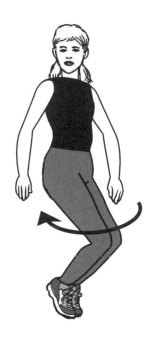

PURPOSE

Improve elastic strength in ankles
Enhance rotational mechanics

PROCEDURE

- Stand in a relaxed position with feet shoulder-width apart.
- Perform ankle jumps, rotating 90 degrees in midair.
- Land and immediately jump back to the starting position.
- Repeat to the other side.
- Do as quickly as possible while trying to maintain a fixed, neutral shoulder position.

Scissor Jumps

Lower-Body Plyometric Drills

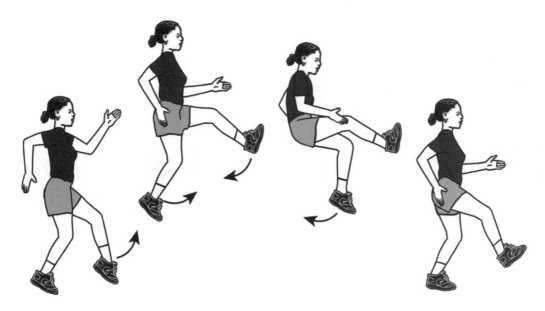

PURPOSE

Improve quickness in hips
Enhance balance

PROCEDURE

- Begin by kicking one leg forward and up into the air as if punting a football.

- While in the air, leave the ground with the opposing leg and repeat with the opposite leg while

the initial leg is returning to the ground.

- Repeat as quickly as possible for a certain amount of reps or for time.

- Make sure you do the equivalent amount of work initiating the drill with the opposite leg.

Quickness

173

Lateral Skaters

Lower-Body Plyometric Drills

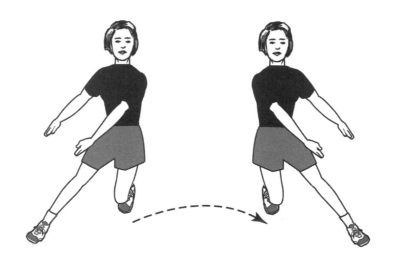

PURPOSE

Improve cutting ability and first-step lateral quickness

PROCEDURE

- Begin with both feet together and push off laterally with one leg.
- Upon landing, immediately push off in the opposite direction and continue the drill for either reps or time.
- To develop quickness, perform as many reps as possible for time (10 seconds or less).

COMPLEX VARIATION

- Jump diagonally so as to move laterally and forward.

In-Place Tuck Jumps

Lower-Body Plyometric Drills

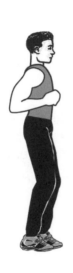
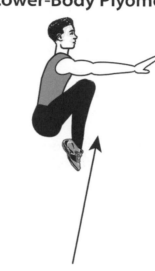

PURPOSE

Improve power in the lower body

PROCEDURE

- Standing in the power position, load the lower body by swinging both arms back while flexing the hips and knees.

- Begin the extension of the hips and knees and finally the ankles as the arms swing forward but close to the body.

- Jump straight in the air tucking both knees to the chest.

- Upon landing, repeat immediately with the same technique.

- For quickness, perform as rapidly as possible for time while counting reps, or for a fixed number of reps as rapidly as possible.

- This drill may be performed with a single leg as well.

COMPLEX VARIATION

- Perform a pike jump, keeping your legs straight while tucking.

Quickness

175

Vertical Jump

Lower-Body Plyometric Drills

PURPOSE

Improve quickness and explosive power in the lower body

PROCEDURE

- Stand with the feet shoulder-width apart (with the knees and hips flexed in a prestretched position and with the arms back and shoulders over the toes) and quickly dip into the "power position."

- Perform a vertical jump by sequentially extending the ankles, knees, and hips, followed by the arms reaching straight up into the air.

COMPLEX VARIATION

- Upon landing, immediately reload the legs and perform another vertical jump sequence, spending as little time as possible on the ground.

Quickness

Standing Long Jump

Lower-Body Plyometric Drills

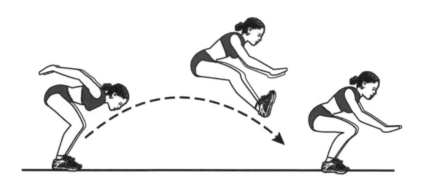

PURPOSE

Improve lower body power

PROCEDURE

- Start standing with both feet about shoulder-width apart or slightly narrower.

- Load the legs by flexing the knees and hips and cocking the arms backward.

- Propel your body up and out for distance by extending the legs and using the arms to help thrust the body forward for distance.

Quickness

177

Barrier Jumps

Lower-Body Plyometric Drills

PURPOSE

Improve power and quickness in the lower body

PROCEDURE

- Using something for a barrier (hurdle, cones, boxes), propel your body over the barrier by jumping forward using an ankle-knee-hip extension.

- Maintaining a vertical body posture, tuck the knees to your chest while clearing the obstacle.

- Use a double-arm swing to maintain balance and assist in achieving vertical height.

COMPLEX VARIATIONS

- Lateral Barrier Jumps—This variation is the same as Barrier Jumps except for the barrier now being conquered laterally. Begin by standing parallel to the barrier. Use the same loading action as described above, but now propel your body over the obstacle laterally. Upon landing, load the legs and arms once again and immediately jump laterally back over the barrier. Continue as quickly as possible for a set amount of jumps or for time.

- Single Leg Barrier Jumps—This variation is the same as Barrier Jumps but with one leg at a time. This adds a great degree of difficulty to the jump and should be performed over shorter obstacles at first with gradual increases in height.

Triple Jump

Lower-Body Plyometric Drills

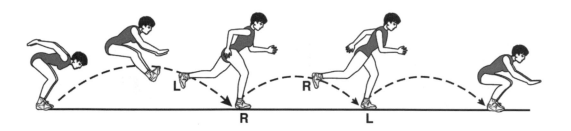

PURPOSE

Improve lower body power and quickness

PROCEDURE

- Perform a long jump and land on one leg.
- Bound to the other leg.
- Bound and land on both feet.

Quickness

179

Plyo to Sprint

Lower-Body Plyometric Drills

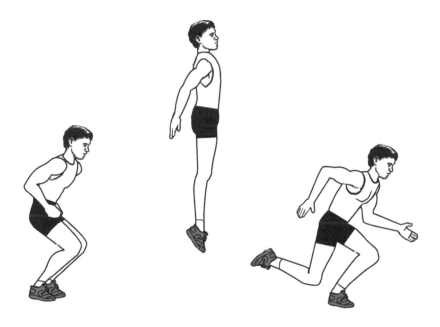

PURPOSE

Improve quickness and power in the lower body

PROCEDURE

- Perform any plyometric exercise and sprint immediately upon landing.
- The plyometric exercise may be stationary or movement-oriented.
- You may perform one or more repetitions before the sprint.
- For example, you may perform three vertical jumps followed by a 20-yard sprint.

COMPLEX VARIATION

- Reverse drill and perform sprint to plyo.

Quickness

REFERENCES

1. Bompa, T. 2000. *Total Training for Young Champions.* United States: Versa Press

2. Bompa, T. 1994. *Power Training for Sport Performance: Plyometrics for Maximum Power Development.* Oakville, New York and London: Mosaic Press.

3. Bompa, T. 1999. *Periodization: Training for Sports.* United States: Versa Press.

4. Chu, D. 1996. *Explosive Power and Strength.* United States: Versa Press.

5. Drabik, J. 1996. *Children & Sports Training.* Island Pond, Vermont: Stadion Publishing Company, Inc.

6. Gambetta, V. 1998. *Soccer Speed.* United States: Gambetta Sports Training Systems.

7. Gambetta, V. and Odgers, S. 1991. *The Complete Guide to Medicine Ball Training.* United States: Optimum Sports Training.

8. Little, J (editor). 1997. *Bruce Lee: Bruce Lee's Commentaries on the Martial Way.* Vol. 3. Boston, Vermont and Tokyo: Charles E. Tuttle Co., Inc.

9. Morgan, G.T. and McGlynn, G. H. 1997. *Cross-Training for Sports.* United States: Versa Press.

10. Siff, M. and Verkhoshansky, Y. 1999. *SUPERTRAINING.* Fourth Ed. Denver USA: Supertraining International.

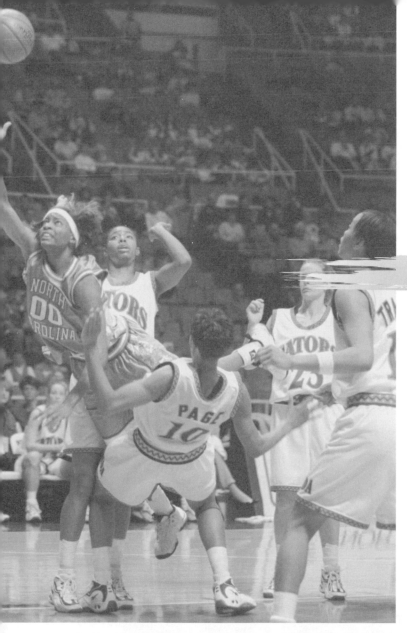

Sport-Specific Speed, Agility, and Quickness Programs

Vance A. Ferrigno, CSCS

Juan Carlos Santana, MS

This chapter is designed to give you examples of how to use the drills in this book. The sport-specific programs emphasize proper progression from basic to complex speed, agility, and quickness drills. These programs are not intended to be a "cookie-cutter" approach to sport-specific program design. Every athlete has distinctive goals and needs, even if the sport and position are the same.

Speed, agility, and quickness drills cover the complete spectrum of biomotor skills, from basic and low intensity to complex and high intensity. Some of the basic skills, like skipping and medicine ball work, can be used in the warm-up section of any training session. Other drills of higher intensity, like jumping drills, can put an enormous stress on physiological structures, as well as the central nervous system (CNS). These higher intensity drills should be used wisely and ample recovery between drills and training sessions should be provided. For safety and variety, limit speed, agility, and quickness training sessions to twice per week, preferably on days when weight training is not performed.

The information derived from the "Needs Analysis" section is the key to properly designing a safe and effective speed, agility, and quickness program. Once you have decided the major goals of the year, several mesocycles can be programmed to more specifically address the objectives of the training program. The programs we have provided are mesocycles geared at improving speed, agility, and quickness in various sports. Each mesocycle consists of 6 microcycles (i.e. 6 weeks). Adjustments can and should always be made to each microcycle to insure the training program stays on track and that consistent safe progress is made.

It is important to note that speed, agility, and quickness training is just one segment of the total training plan, which also includes functional strength, balance, flexibility, and proper restoration. Each one of these may be your emphasis depending on where you are in your athletic development or training cycle. For the purpose of this chapter we will assume that the major emphasis for the current mesocycle is speed, agility, and quickness training. We will also assume that basic locomotive mechanics have been mastered and that the general preparation phase has been completed.

There are many variables in designing a training program. Although we may show one drill to be performed twice in one week, if the skill is mastered easily a more complex variation can be attempted to maintain progress. The first three weeks are dedicated to mastering specific skills. In the second three weeks of the mesocycle, we mix and match several drills to create complex drills. Here is the time to get creative with your program. Feel free to change a drill, combine it with a sport-specific skill, or combine it with another drill. Experimentation is how all of these drills were developed. However, it is important to make sure that the basic movement patterns are mastered before increasing their complexity or combining with another skill. A complex drill done sloppily will do more harm than good because it will create a poor motor program.

The session format can be tailored to meet the specific needs and goals of the athlete, or the team as a whole.

- 3-5 minute session introduction: Lay out the main goals of the session
- 10 minute warm-up
- Body of session: 20-25 sets of drills with a 1:3-1:4 work to rest ratio
- Provide several 3-minute breaks for water, especially in hot climates
- 5-minute flexibility exercises and positive reflections of the session

After the introduction to the session, begin the preparation with a dynamic warm-up. As the drills of a session are mastered, they can eventually be used in the warm-up. Many of the drills in this book, such as skipping and carioca, can serve as warm-up exercises. Using simple speed, agility, and quickness drills in the warm-up serves two main objectives. First, it prepares the body and CNS for work. Second, it teaches and reinforces proper biomotor skill execution, without taking time away from the main goal of the training session. A 10-minute warm-up, over the course of a mesocycle (i.e. 20 minutes per week, 2 hours per mesocycle), can have a profound effect on biomotor skill acquisition and conditioning.

Use the following guidelines to insure a safe and effective progression in the warm-up and during the entire training cycle.

- Simple drills / Complex drills
- Slow execution speeds / Fast execution speeds
- Low intensity drills / High intensity drills
- Correct execution / Higher volumes and intensities

Below is a sample of a 10-minute warm-up using the drills in this book. Perform each drill 2-4 times over 15-20 yards.

- "A" march (to knee hug)
- "B" march
- Light jog
- Back pedal
- Skip with relaxed arm swing
- Backward skip with relaxed arm swing
- Straight leg shuffle
- Backward straight leg shuffle
- Side shuffle with relaxed arm swing
- Carioca
- Stand up from four points

The body of the session can emphasize the major weaknesses of an athlete or group. It isn't necessary to perform an even number of sets for each drill. If a particular drill is providing a challenge, focus on that drill over ones that have been mastered. Prioritize drills with those that require more emphasis at the beginning of the session followed by those which provide maintenance. Provide ample rest between each drill. Remember that the focus is to develop speed, agility, and quickness. This development cannot take place in a fatigued state. A 1:3-1:4 work to rest ratio should provide ample rest. However, if your athletes are not well-conditioned, they may need more time for recovery. In this case, lower the sets per session and increase the rest periods, and you'll get more out of the session with this approach. More is not always better. When using speed, agility, and quickness training for conditioning, try to match the work-to-rest ratio or training to the work-to-rest ratio of the target sport in order to make training metabolically specific to the sport.

Because of individual differences, specific recommendations on the volume and intensity of exercises are impossible to make. However, ranges may be provided to serve as general guidelines. Exercises which involve jumping and throwing medicine balls can be performed 5-10 times per set, depending on intensity and the athlete's level of conditioning. Exercises involving hard-surface contact, such as explosive push-ups, punching, slide exercises, and side strike drills, can be performed 10-15 times each. Tumbling exercises can be performed 3-5 times per set. Running patterns are performed once per set and the distance should be specific to the target sport. All exercises can be performed for the maximum number that can be accomplished in a specified period of time, usually between 5 and 10 seconds. This approach to short, intense intervals provides high intensity biomotor development and excellent metabolic conditioning.

Water breaks are a great way to provide rest and well-needed nourishment to the body, especially in hot climates. Keep water close by and provide breaks after the warm-up, in the middle of the main body of the session, and at the end of the main body of the session (i.e. before flexibility work). Athletes are not very conscientious about hydrating properly before a training session; therefore, you are better off to make sure they are hydrated properly.

The flexibility session is a time of gearing down, working on range-of-motion (ROM) issues, and positively reflecting on the session. This is the time to use static flexibility, but should not turn into a flexibility contest. Rather it should focus on individual ROM issues and the maintenance of healthy ROM.

Finish every session with positive affirmations. Focus on the success of the session, not the failures. Speak of needed improvements in a positive manner and communicate an eagerness to accomplish your goals. No athlete or team likes to be reminded of their shortcomings. Your athletes will respond better to a positive and respectful coaching style. Developing a good work ethic and desire to perform at the highest level possible begins with mutual respect and admiration, in the coach and the athlete.

GOALS
Improve serving power, change of direction, and reaction time

NEEDS	WEEK 1 Drill name	#	WEEK 2 Drill name	#	WEEK 3 Drill name	#
Speed	Ankling	3	"A" Skip for Distance (v)	9	"A" Skip for Height (v)	9
	Wall Drills (Acceleration Marches)	34	Falling Starts	35	Heavy Sled Pulls	44
Agility	Icky Shuffle	68	Carioca	69	In-Out Shuffle	70
	20-Yard Shuttle	57	T-Drill	58	15-Yard Turn Drill	61
Quickness	Side Shuffle	115	Lateral Skaters	173	Lateral Skaters to Sprint	173 -179
	MB Wall Scoop Toss	146	MB Side-to-Side Pass (v)	144	MB Wall Overhead Throw	145

NEEDS	WEEK 4 Drill name	#	WEEK 5 Drill name	#	WEEK 6 Drill name	#
Speed, agility, and quickness	Zigzag	74	Crossover Shuffle	73	Zigzag Crossover Shuffle	75
	Lateral 20-Yard Shuttle (v)	57	Sprint and Cut on Command	151	8-point Star Drill	153
Speed and quickness	Sprint to MB Wall Side Toss	179 -144	MB Overhead Throw to Sprint	145 -179	Side Shuffle to MB Side-to-Side Pass (v)	115 -144
	Quick Feet	159	Hop-Scotch Drill	164	Half Ladder Skill While Climbing (v)	168
Agility and quickness	Side-to-Side With Cone Reach	89	Side-to-Side While Catching (v)	89	Side-to-Side While Volleying (v)	89

Note:
(v) = variation

Comments:
_____

_____

_____

_____

_____

_____

_____

_____

GOALS

Defense: Increased vertical jump for blocks; Improve reaction and level changes for digs; Improve lateral quickness for digs. Offense: Improve vertical jump and core for spiking

NEEDS	WEEK 1 Drill name	#	WEEK 2 Drill name	#	WEEK 3 Drill name	#
Speed	Standing Stationary Arm Swings	1	Weighted Arm Swings (v)	1	Contrast Resisted Arm Swings (v)	1
	Straight Leg Shuffle	4	"A" Skips	9	Skipping for Height (v)	9
Agility	Forward Roll	98	Backward Roll	99	Sprawl and Stand Up	97
	Carioca	55	Side-to-Side With Cone Reach	89	Side-to-Side With Volley (v)	89
Quickness	Hip-Twist Ankle Jumps	171	In-Place Tuck Jumps	174	Pike Jumps (v)	174
	MB Wall Chest Passes	141	Tap Drills	125	One-Handed Tap Drills With Partner	126

NEEDS	WEEK 4 Drill name	#	WEEK 5 Drill name	#	WEEK 6 Drill name	#
Speed , agility, and quickness	Foot-Tapping Frequency to Bounce and Catch	147 -135	Side Shuffle to Bounce and Catch	115 -135	Side Shuffle to Sprawl and Stand Up	115 -97
	Stand Up From Four Points	94	Stand Up From a Sitting Position	95	Stand Up From a Lying Position (v)	96
Speed and quickness	MB Overhead Throw to Sprint	145 -179	MB Overhead Throw to Vertical Jump	145 -175	MB Overhead Throw to Sprint	145 -179
	Repeated Vertical Jumps (v)	175	Side Shuffle to Quick Hands Toss	115 -133	Side Shuffle to Ball Drops	115 -132
Agility and quickness	Backward Roll to Vertical Jump	99 -175	Forward Roll to Vertical Jump	98 -175	Sprawl and Stand Up to Vertical Jump	97 -175
	Side Shuffle to Quick Hands Toss	115 -133	Lateral Skaters to Bounce and Catch	173 -135	Lateral Skaters to Quick Hands	173 -133

Note:
(v) = variation

Comments:

_____

_____

_____

_____

_____

_____

_____

_____

GOALS
Rotational power for punching and kicking; Quickness for body positioning; Quickness in hand and eye coordination and reaction

NEEDS	WEEK 1 Drill name	#	WEEK 2 Drill name	#	WEEK 3 Drill name	#
Speed	Skip for Height	50	Skip for Distance (v)	51	Split-Squat Jumps	52
	Stadium Stairs	42	Uphill Acceleration Run	43	Heavy Sled Pulls	44
Agility	Icky Shuffle	68	Carioca	69	In-Out Shuffle	70
	One Side Skier	87	5-Dot Drill	110	Flip and Catch	111
Quickness	Rope-Skipping	169	Hip-Twist Ankle Jumps	171	Scissor Jumps	172
	The Bob	120	The Parry	121	The Weave	122

NEEDS	WEEK 4 Drill name	#	WEEK 5 Drill name	#	WEEK 6 Drill name	#
Speed, agility, and quickness	Running Balance (v)	2	Running Balance (v)	2	Running Balance (v)	2
	Snake Jumps	76	180-Degree Turn	77	Slalom Ski Jump	78
Speed and quickness	Boxing Focus Mitt Simple Drills	123	Boxing Focus Mitt Complex Drills	124	The Bob to Boxing Focus Mitt Simple Drills	120 -123
	The Bob to The Weave	120 -122	The Parry to The Weave	121 -122	The Weave to Boxing Focus Complex Drills	122 -124
Agility and quickness	Plyo Push-Ups	140	MB Wall Chest Passes	141	Single-Arm MB Chest Pass (v)	141
	Forward Roll to Scissor Jumps	98 -172	Backward Roll to Vertical Jump	99 -175	Cartwheel to Barrier Jump	102 -177

Note:
(v) = variation

Comments:

_____

_____

_____

_____

_____

_____

_____

GOALS

Explosive power; Powerful rotational mechanics for throws; Agility from athletic position and quick reaction

NEEDS	WEEK 1 Drill name	#	WEEK 2 Drill name	#	WEEK 3 Drill name	#
Speed	"A" Skips	9	"A" Runs (v)	9	Sand Running	25
	Stadium Stairs	42	Uphill Acceleration Run	43	Heavy Sled Pull	44
Agility	Forward Roll/ Backward Roll	101	Sprawl and Stand Up	97	Sprawl, Roll, and Stand Up (v)	97
	Snake Jumps	76	180-Degree Turn	77	Bag Jumps with 180-Degree Turn	83
Quickness	Wheelbarrow	139	Stability Ball Hops	138	Medicine Ball Punches	143
	Weighted Rope Skipping (v)	169	In-Place Tuck Jumps	174	Repeated Pike Jumps (v)	174

NEEDS	WEEK 4 Drill name	#	WEEK 5 Drill name	#	WEEK 6 Drill name	#
Speed, agility, and quickness	Dodge Ball	134	Dodge Ball to Sprawl and Stand Up	134 -97	Dodge Ball to Tuck Jumps	134 -174
	The Bob	120	The Parry	121	The Weave	122
Speed and quickness	MB Wall Side Toss	144	MB Overhead Throw	145	MB Scoop Reverse Toss (v)	146
	Repeated Vertical Jumps (v)	175	Split-Squat Jumps	52	Alternating Split-Squat Jumps (v)	52
Agility and quickness	Cross-Behind Step	86	One Side Skier	87	Side-to-Side Skiers	88
	Sprawl and Stand Up to MB Punches	97 -143	Sprawl and Stand Up to Vertical Jump	97 -175	Sprawl and Stand Up to Barrier Jump	97 -177

Note:
(v) = variation

Comments:

_____

_____

_____

_____

_____

_____

_____

_____

BASEBALL, SOFTBALL, AND CRICKET—Infielders   *Sample Program*

GOALS
Quick response and lateral movement for throwing speed and fielding range; Acceleration and turning ability for faster base running; Increased bat speed

NEEDS	WEEK 1 Drill name	#	WEEK 2 Drill name	#	WEEK 3 Drill name	#
Speed	"A" Skips	9	Light Sled/Tire Pulls	21	Parachute Running	24
	Wall Drills (Acceleration Marches)	34	Acceleration Runs	40	Uphill Acceleration Run	43
Agility	20-Yard Shuttle	57	Figure Eights	64	Z-Pattern Run	65
	Zigzag	74	Crossover Shuffle	73	Zigzag Crossover Shuffle	75
Quickness	Ball Drops with a Partner	132	Bounce and Catch	135	Goalie Drill	136
	MB Overhead Throw	145	MB Wall Side Toss	144	MB Side-to-Side (v)	144

NEEDS	WEEK 4 Drill name	#	WEEK 5 Drill name	#	WEEK 6 Drill name	#
Speed, agility, and quickness	Side-to-Side with Cone Reach	89	Side-to-Side with Front Rotation	91	Side-to-Side with Back Rotation	92
	15-Yard Turn Drill	61	20-Yard Square	62	30-Yard Square (v)	62
Speed and quickness	Side Shuffle	154	Back Shuffle	156	Sprint and Cut on Command	151
	Sprint to MB Overhead Throw	179 -145	Sprint to MB Side Toss	179 -144	MB Side Toss to Sprint	144 -179
Agility and quickness	180-Degree Turn	77	Slalom Ski Jump	78	Lateral Skaters	173
	Icky Shuffle While Fielding Ball (v)	68	Crossover Shuffle While Fielding (v)	73	Half-Ladder Skill to Pick Up Ball (v)	167

Note:
(v) = variation

Comments:

_____

_____

_____

_____

_____

_____

_____

GOALS
First-step quickness; Acceleration; Change of direction

NEEDS	WEEK 1 Drill name	#	WEEK 2 Drill name	#	WEEK 3 Drill name	#
Speed	Straight Leg Shuffle	4	Single-Leg Run Through	17	Run Through	18
	Wall Drills (Acceleration Marches)	34	Uphill Acceleration Run	43	Heavy Sled Pulls	44
Agility	Stand Up from 4 Points	94	Squirm	59	Squirm (v)	59
	15-Yard Turn Drill	61	Z-Pattern Cuts	67	Change of Direction	79
Quickness	Plyo Push-Ups	140	Stability Ball Cyclic Impact Lockouts	137	Stability Ball Hops	138
	MB Wall Chest Passes	141	Two-Arm MB Wall Chest Passes (v)	141	One-Arm MB Punches (v)	143

NEEDS	WEEK 4 Drill name	#	WEEK 5 Drill name	#	WEEK 6 Drill name	#
Speed, agility, and quickness	Crossover Step	85	Cross-Behind Step	86	One Side Skier	87
	Bag Weave	80	Lateral Weave	82	Bag Jumps with 180-Degree Turn	83
Speed and quickness	One-Arm MB Punch to Sprint	143 -179	Sprint to One-Arm MB Punch	179 -143	Sprint to Plyo Variation (v)	179
	MB Wall Scoop Toss	146	MB Squat, Push Toss, Bounce, and Catch	130	MB Reverse Scoop Toss, Bounce, and Catch	131
Agility and quickness	Forward Roll to Ball Catch (v)	98	Sprint to Forward Roll	179 -98	Running Start and Tumbling Over Barrier	104
	Stand Up From Four Points to Ball Catch (v)	94	Sprawl and Stand Up to Ball Catch (v)	97	Sprawl and Stand Up to Sprint (v)	97 -179

Note:
(v) = variation

Comments:
_____
_____
_____
_____
_____
_____
_____
_____
_____

GOALS

Defense: Improve jumping ability for rebounding and blocking; Improve lateral mobility for coverage and change of direction. Offense: Improve jumping ability for shooting; Improve first-step quickness and acceleration for breakaways

NEEDS	WEEK 1 Drill name	#	WEEK 2 Drill name	#	WEEK 3 Drill name	#
Speed	"A" March Walk	8	"A" Skip for Distance (v)	9	"A" Skip for Height (v)	9
	"A" Form Runs (v)	9	Partner-Resisted Starts	45	Bullet Belt	49
Agility	20-Yard Shuttle	57	Lateral 20-Yard Shuttle (v)	57	T-Drill	58
	MB Wall Chest Passes	141	MB Overhead Throw	145	MB Wall Scoop Toss	146
Quickness	Repeated Vertical Jumps (v)	175	Standing Long Jump	176	Triple Jump	178

NEEDS	WEEK 4 Drill name	#	WEEK 5 Drill name	#	WEEK 6 Drill name	#
Speed, agility, and quickness	Squirm	59	X-Pattern Multi-Skill	63	Z-Pattern Cuts	67
	Hexagon Drill	109	5-Dot Drill	110	21 Drill	106
Speed and quickness	Quick Feet	159	Hop Scotch Drill to Catch a Pass (v)	164	One-Leg Hop to Dribble and Lay-up (v)	165
	Repeated Vertical Jumps (v)	175	Vertical Jump to Sprint	175-179	Sprint to Vertical Jump	179-175
Agility and quickness	Tap Drills	125	MB Lateral Shuffle/Pass	128	Mirror Lateral Shuffle/Pass	129
	Stand Up From 4 Points to 20-Yard Shuttle	94-57	Stand Up From Sitting Position to Z-Pattern Run	95-65	Stand Up From Lying Position to T-Drill	96-58

Note:
(v) = variation

Comments:

_____

_____

_____

_____

_____

_____

_____

_____

_____

GOALS

Improve explosive power and quickness for faster dash times

NEEDS	WEEK 1 Drill name	#	WEEK 2 Drill name	#	WEEK 3 Drill name	#
Speed	Running Balance	2	Ankling	3	"A" Skip	9
	Wall Drills (Acceleration Marches)	34	Falling Starts	35	Acceleration Runs	40
	[Basic 40-yard Model	37	Gears	38	Ins and Outs	39
Agility	20-yard Shuttle	57	Carioca	69	Crossover Skipping	56
Quickness	In-Place Ankle Jumps	170	In-Place Tuck Jumps One-Arm MB Punch	174 -143	Standing Long Jump	176
	MB Wall Chest Passes	141	Chest Pass (v)	141	MB Wall Side Toss	144

NEEDS	WEEK 4 Drill name	#	WEEK 5 Drill name	#	WEEK 6 Drill name	#
Speed, agility, and quickness	Seated Arm Swings (v)	1	Seated Weighted Arm Swings (v)	1	Contrast Resisted Arm Swings (v)	1
	"B" Skips	12	Uphill Speed Runs	22	Partner Tubing-Assisted Speed Runs	30
Speed and quickness	Weighted Starts	41	Partner-Assisted Let-Go's	48	Partner Tubing-Assisted Acceleration Drill	46
	Side-to-Side with Cone Reach	89	Front to Back	90	Side-to-Side with Front and Back Rotation	93
Agility and quickness	Barrier Jumps	177	Triple Jump	178	Plyo to Sprint	179
	MB Overhead Throw	145	MB Wall Scoop Toss	146	MB Squat, Push Toss, Bounce, and Catch	130

Note:
(v) = variation

Comments:

_____

_____

_____

_____

_____

_____

SOCCER AND LACROSSE—Strikers and Forwards   *Sample Program*

GOALS
Lateral agility and quickness; Level changes during slide tackles; Open field acceleration

NEEDS	WEEK 1 Drill name	#	WEEK 2 Drill name	#	WEEK 3 Drill name	#
Speed	Single-Leg Run Through	17	Run Through	18	Run Through Alternating Fast Legs (v)	18
	Gears	38	Uphill Speed Runs	22	Uphill-to-Flat Contrast Speed Runs	27
Agility	Figure Eights	64	Z-Pattern Run	65	Z-Pattern Cuts	67
	Stand Up From Four Points	94	Sprawl and Stand Up	97	Sprawl, Roll, and Stand Up (v)	97
Quickness	Skips to Reaction Sprint (v)	160	Side Step to Reaction Sprint (v)	161	Change of Skill to Reaction Sprint (v)	166
	Repeated Vertical Jumps (v)	175	Lateral Skaters	173	Vertical Jump to Sprint	175 -179

NEEDS	WEEK 4 Drill name	#	WEEK 5 Drill name	#	WEEK 6 Drill name	#
Speed, agility, and quickness	Stand Up From Four Points to 20-Yard Shuttle	94 -57	Sprawl and Stand Up to Squirm	97 -59	Forward Roll/Backward Roll to Squirm	101 -59
	Forward Roll	98	Backward Roll	99	Cartwheel	102
Speed and quickness	MB Overhead Throw	145	MB Wall Scoop Toss	146	MB Squat, Push Toss, Bounce, and	130
	Lateral Skaters	173	Repeated Vertical Jumps (v)	175	Sprint to Vertical Jump	179 -175
Agility and quickness	Half Ladder Skill to Ball Control (v)	167	Half Ladder Skill to Shoot (v)	167	Half Ladder Skill to Trap and Shoot (v)	167
	Sprint and Backpedal on Command	150	Sprint and Cut on Command	151	8-Point Star Drill	153

Note:
 (v) = variation

Comments:

_____

_____

_____

_____

_____

GOALS

NEEDS	WEEK 1 Drill name	#	WEEK 2 Drill name	#	WEEK 3 Drill name	#
Speed						
Agility						
Quickness						

NEEDS	WEEK 4 Drill name	#	WEEK 5 Drill name	#	WEEK 6 Drill name	#
Speed, agility, and quickness						
Speed and quickness						
Agility and quickness						

Note:
(v) = variation

Comments:

_____

_____

_____

_____

_____

_____

Drill List

Acceleration Ladder (Stick) Drills

40. Acceleration Runs (17- and 4-inch)

Resisted Acceleration Drills

41. Weighted Starts
42. Stadium Stairs
43. Uphill Acceleration Run
44. Heavy Sled Pulls
45. Partner-Resisted Starts

Assisted Acceleration Drills

46. Partner Tubing-Assisted Acceleration Drill
47. Towed Running (Pulley)

Contrast Acceleration Drills

48. Partner-Assisted Let-Go's
49. Bullet Belt

Plyometric Drills

50. Skip for Height
51. Skip for Distance
52. Split-Squat Jumps
53. Bounding
54. Single-Leg Bounds

AGILITY DRILLS .. p.85

Assorted Biomotor Skills

55. Carioca
56. Crossover Skipping

Line Drills

57. 20-Yard Shuttle (Pro Agility)
58. T-Drill
59. Squirm
60. 40-Yard Ladder Sprint

Cone Drills

61. 15-Yard Turn Drill
62. 20-Yard Square
63. X-Pattern Multi-Skill
64. Figure Eights

65. Z-Pattern Run
66. Zigzag
67. Z-Pattern Cuts

Agility Ladder Drills

68. Icky Shuffle
69. Carioca
70. In-Out Shuffle
71. Side Right-In
72. Side Left-In
73. Crossover Shuffle
74. Zigzag
75. Zigzag Crossover Shuffle
76. Snake Jump
77. 180-Degree Turn
78. Slalom Ski Jump

Bag Drills

79. Change of Direction
80. Bag Weave
81. Combo Side Step/Forward Back
82. Lateral Weave
83. Bag Jumps with 180-Degree Turn
84. Wheel

Angle-Board Drills

85. Crossover Step
86. Cross-Behind Step
87. One Side Skiers
88. Side-to-Side Skiers

Slide Board Drills

89. Side-to-Side With Cone Reach
90. Front to Back
91. Side-to-Side With Front Rotation
92. Side-to-Side With Back Rotation
93. Side-to-Side With Front and Back Combination

Level Change Drills

Reactive Stand-Up Drills

94. Stand Up From Four Points
95. Stand Up From a Sitting Position
96. Stand Up From a Lying Position
97. Sprawl and Stand Up

Tumbling Drills

98. Forward Roll Over Shoulder
99. Backward Roll Over Shoulder
100. Backward Roll to Hand Push-Off
101. Forward Roll/ Backward Roll Combination
102. Cartwheel
103. Round-Off
104. Running Start and Tumbling Over Barrier
105. Tumbling Sequencing

Miscellaneous Crazy Z-Ball Drills

106. Z-Ball 21 Drill
107. Drop and Get Up
108. Under and Go

Hex and Dot Drills

109. Hexagon Drill
110. 5-Dot Drill

Medicine Ball Drills

111. Flip and Catch
112. Toss, Get Up, and Catch

QUICKNESS DRILLS p.151

Assorted Biomotor Skills

113. Backpedal
114. Multi-Directional Skipping
115. Side Shuffle

Reaction Drills

116. Reaction Arm Sprints
117. Hot Hands
118. Card Release
119. Card Snatching

Defensive Boxing Drills

120. The Bob (Slip)
121. The Parry (Slap Block)
122. The Weave

Offensive Boxing Drills

123. Boxing Focus Mitt Simple Drills
124. Boxing Focus Mitt Complex Drills

Medicine Ball Reaction Drills

125. Tap Drills (Simple Reaction Touches to a Target on Command)
126. One-Handed Tap Drills With Partner
127. Medicine Ball Bull in a Ring
128. Medicine Ball Lateral Shuffle/Pass
129. Mirror Lateral Shuffle/Pass
130. Medicine Ball Squat, Push Toss, Bounce, and Catch
131. Medicine Ball Reverse Scoop Toss, Bounce, and Catch

Sports Ball Reaction Drills

132. Ball Drops With a Partner
133. Quick Hands Toss
134. Dodge Ball
135. Bounce and Catch
136. Goalie Drill (Line Creates Boundary)
137. Stability Ball Cyclic Impact Lockouts
138. Stability Ball Hops

Upper-Body Plyometric Drills

139. Wheelbarrow Drill
140. Plyo Push-Ups
141. Medicine Ball Wall Chest Passes
142. Medicine Ball Release Push-Ups With Partner
143. Medicine Ball Punches
144. Medicine Ball Wall Side Toss
145. Medicine Ball Overhead Throw
146. Medicine Ball Wall Scoop Toss

Lower-Body Reaction Drills

147. Foot-Tapping Frequency
148. Directional Foot Movement
149. Directional Mirror Drill

Reactive Running Drills

150. Sprint and Backpedal on Command
151. Sprint and Cut on Command

152. Backpedal and Cut on Command
153. 8-Point Star Drill

Angle-Board Drills

154. Side Shuffle
155. Front Shuffle
156. Back Shuffle

Medicine Ball Explosive Drills

157. Medicine Ball Between Leg Flips (Maravich)
158. Pike Kick Up and Catch

Half Agility Ladder Drills With Reaction Command

159. Quick Feet (in All Directions)
160. Skips
161. Side Step
162. Side Step/Double Step
163. Bunny Jumps
164. Hop-Scotch Drill

165. One-Leg Hop
166. Change of Skill
167. Half Ladder Skill to Sport-Specific Skill
168. Half Ladder Skill While Performing Sport-Specific Activity

Lower-Body Plyometric Drills

169. Rope-Skipping
170. In-Place Ankle Jumps
171. Hip-Twist Ankle Jumps
172. Scissor Jumps
173. Lateral Skaters
174. In-Place Tuck Jumps
175. Vertical Jump
176. Standing Long Jump
177. Barrier Jumps
178. Triple Jump
179. Plyo to Sprint

Editors

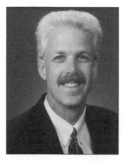

Lee E. Brown is a certified strength and conditioning specialist (CSCS) through the National Strength and Conditioning Association (NSCA) and is on the NSCA board of directors. He is also a certified health fitness instructor through the American College of Sports Medicine (ACSM) and a certified club coach by USA Weightlifting Federation (USAWF). Brown holds a master's degree in exercise science and a doctorate in educational leadership from Florida Atlantic University. Formerly a high school physical education teacher and coach of many sports, Brown now teaches advanced strength and conditioning courses and serves as assistant professor and director of the Human Performance Laboratory at Arkansas State University. He lives in Jonesboro, Arkansas.

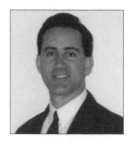

Vance Ferrigno is a certified strength & conditioning specialist with the NSCA and serves on the NSCA Conference Committee. He is also certified through ACSM as a health/fitness director & health/fitness instructor, and is a USAWF Club Coach. Ferrigno, who earned his bachelor's degree in exercise science from Florida State University, assists in developing and teaching the curriculum for strength and conditioning at Florida Atlantic University. Ferrigno is currently the Director of Fitness & Aquatics at Woodfield Country Club in Boca Raton, Florida. He resides in Coconut Creek, Florida.

(continued)

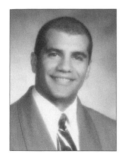

Juan Carlos Santana holds a master's degree in exercise science from Florida Atlantic University and is working on his PhD in exercise physiology at the University of Miami. He is certified by the NSCA (CSCS) and the ACSM (HFI). Santana also holds coaching certifications with USA Weightlifting and USA Track and Field. He is a member of the NSCA Conference Committee and chairs the NSCA Sports Specific Conference. Santana has been a national competitor and coach in five different sports throughout his 20-year athletic and coaching career. He now lectures internationally and directs Optimum Performance Systems, a Florida company that consults for various equipment companies, athletic teams, and private clients. Santana lives in Boca Raton, Florida.

Contributors

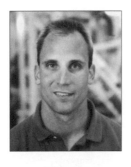

John F. Graham is a CSCS, ACSM-certified health fitness instructor, and USA Weightlifting Level I coach. He is currently pursuing a master of science degree in health and physical education at East Stroudsburg University. Graham has contributed, either as author, coauthor, or expert source, to 85 publications regarding health, fitness, and sport conditioning. He coordinates, designs, and implements exercise prescriptions for athletes and people with chronic diseases and disabilities in his position as director of the Human Performance Center at the Allentown Sports Medicine & Human Performance Center. Currently, he serves as the strength coach and consultant for the U.S. national sprint cycling team and Parkettes gymnastics team.

Andrew Hardyk, MS, assistant track coach at Penn State, is entering his seventh year on the Nittany Lion staff. His responsibilities have increased with his experience: he now coaches the long, high, and triple jumpers, sprinters and hurdlers, and he coordinates the relay team. He has coached three athletes to All-American honors on seven occasions—John Gorham (3), George Audu (3), and Steve Pina (1)—all in the long jump. Hardyk has also coached additional NCAA qualifiers 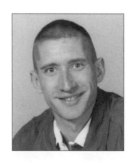 John Whelan (110HH and 55HH), Damon Reed (100m), Phil Oxendine (100m), and Ryan Olkowski (long jump). Hardyk received his bachelor's degree in aerospace engineering in 1992 and a master's degree in engineering mechanics the following year from the University of Cincinnati. He is currently working on his doctorate in sports biomechanics at Penn State.

(continued)

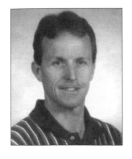

Doug Lentz, CSCS, received a bachelor of science degree from Penn State University in 1981 and has been involved in the conditioning of amateur and professional athletes from high school to postcollegiate levels for almost 20 years. Lentz became a CSCS with the NSCA in 1988. He is a USA Weightlifting Level I coach and has completed work and national testing for the USA Weightlifting Senior Coaches Course. Lentz has also been a member of the editorial board for the American Running Association for over 10 years. He was a faculty member for the first two NSCA Coaches College programs offered in York, Pennsylvania, in 1998 and 1999, and will be a faculty member for the Summer 2000 Coaches College in Carlisle, Pennsylvania. Currently Lentz is the director of fitness and wellness for Chambersburg Health Services (a division of Summit Health) in Chambersburg, Pennsylvania.

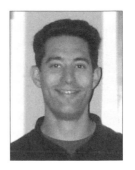

Joshua M. Miller earned his bachelor and master of science degrees at Florida Atlantic University. He holds certifications as a personal trainer with the NSCA, a health fitness instructor with the ACSM, and a club coach with USA Weightlifting Federation. Miller is currently employed as a research graduate assistant at FAU and as an exercise physiologist at Broward General Hospital. He also works as a personal trainer in clients' homes.

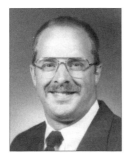

Steven Scott Plisk, MS, CSCS, has been the director of sport conditioning at Yale University since 1997. He received his bachelor of science degree in sport and exercise science from SUNY-Buffalo in 1987 and his master of science degree in kinesiology from the University of Colorado in 1990. He is a CSCS through the NSCA and a Level I coach through USA Weightlifting Federation. His current professional positions include vice president of the NSCA board of directors, associate editor of the *Strength & Conditioning Journal*, faculty member at NSCA Coaches' College, chapter author, and symposium presenter of the NSCA Certification Commission.

Ian Pyka is entering his second year as head strength and conditioning coach for the NHL Florida Panthers. Pyka worked in the same capacity for the University of Massachusetts, Tulane University, and the NFL's New England Patriots before starting his own fitness company in South Florida. He holds a master's degree in exercise physiology from the University of Tennessee and is certified by the NSCA as a CSCS. Pyka was also a three-time All-American and qualified for the 1980 U.S. 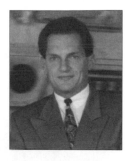 Olympic track and field team as an alternate in the shot put. He has been working as a consultant for clinics and publications dealing with various topics in strength and conditioning for almost two decades. He has published numerous articles in the field of fitness and sport conditioning and has helped produce several training videos.

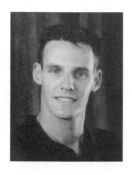

Jim Roberts received his master of science degree in exercise physiology from Florida Atlantic University. He is a CSCS through the NSCA, a specialist in the biomechanics of resistance training through the Cooper Institute for Aerobic Research, and holds a club coach certification from the USA Weightlifting Federation. He is currently a master trainer for the Athletic Club Boca Raton in Boca Raton, Florida, where he specializes in functional assessment and functional strength and conditioning. Roberts' knowledge, coupled with his experience in the field of sports medicine, gives him a truly unique approach of merging the sound principles of biomechanics with dynamic functional life movements that optimize human performance.

Diane Vives, CSCS, received her bachelor's degree in exercise science and wellness from Florida Atlantic University. She is actively involved in several ongoing video projects as well as the USA Weightlifting Federation (USAWF) certification processes. Vives is a member and a certified health fitness instructor with the ACSM and a member and CSCS with the NSCA. She is also a certified club coach with USAWF. Vives is currently the director of operations and video productions for OPS, a 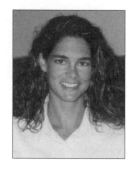 performance enhancement consulting company based in Boca Raton, Florida. Vives focuses on balanced athletic development with an emphasis on functional strength development. She presents on these topics of athletic development and regularly assists OPS in all its presentations provided to top organizations such as the NSCA, USTA, and USAWF.

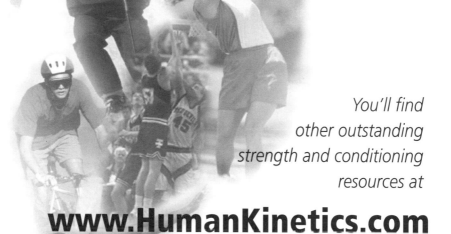